The Community Health Worker

Working guide
Guidelines for training
Guidelines for adaptation

World Health Organization
Geneva
1987

ISBN 92 4 156097 5

Printed in England
85/6659–Clays–10000

Contents

Contents

Part 2 Guidelines for training community health workers

Part 3 Guidelines for adapting this book

Preface

This guide was originally issued in 1974 as a WHO working document entitled "Training and utilization of village health workers". That document was extensively field-tested, and in 1977 it was published as an experimental edition entitled "The primary health worker". The book proved very successful and stocks were rapidly exhausted. In 1980, the experimental edition was further modified in the light of more information from the users, and a revised edition was issued in five languages: Arabic, English, French, Spanish, and Russian. Since then, adaptations and/or translations have been published in many countries.

The present book is a completely revised and enlarged version of the 1980 publication. Apart from improvements and additions to the technical content, the reader will find in this edition clearer illustrations, larger print, and improved layout and presentation of the text and drawings. These changes were deemed necessary in view of the experience gained from the use of the previous version and the demand for better learning materials for community health workers.

It is emphasized, however, that this book is designed for adaptation to local conditions. To help national health authorities in preparing local editions of the learning material given in the working guide (Part 1), the final part of this book contains guidelines for adaptation.

As all learning material has to be regularly updated to suit changing health needs at the local level, WHO welcomes comments on this book from all users. It is hoped that such comments and suggestions will lead to further refinement of the learning material.

Bear in mind that:

This book is intended not only as a learning and reference tool for the community health worker but also as a guide for his or her teacher(s), for those in charge of primary health care programmes, and, more generally, for anyone providing primary health care at family or community levels.

The problems, the text and the drawings should be **adapted** to the conditions of each country and each community in which the community health workers serve. Guidelines for this purpose are given in Part 3 at the end of this book.

Introduction

Countries had been developing their own health services and training their health manpower long before the creation of the World Health Organization (WHO). However, only in a few countries have health services attained wide population coverage. In many, the services benefit mainly urban populations, and the professional health workers who have been trained in the cities tend to stay in the cities and are often not prepared to move to the rural areas to meet the rural people's basic health care needs. In many instances, large hospitals absorb most of a country's health budget, leaving very little for essential primary health care.

The Member States of WHO have gradually come to realize that the provision of sophisticated hospitals and of highly trained staff is not the most efficient way of improving health. Many are now making a big effort to bring more rationality and equity to the development of health services. Consequently, they are placing emphasis on *health* rather than *disease*, and on *health care* rather than *medical care*. In addition, they are giving public health the same attention as individual care.

The notion of basic health services was advocated in the 1960s, and at first it appeared promising. However, reliance on pilot or small-scale projects not adapted to local conditions; and lack of community participation and consequently of local support and resources, resulted in disappointments and failures. Then it became known that the health of the Chinese people had improved spectacularly as a result of what we now call the primary health care approach. One of its guiding principles was the utilization of community health workers (CHWs) to: (*a*) extend health services to the places where the people live and work; (*b*) support communities in identifying their own health needs; and (*c*) help people to solve their own health problems. This new idea that communities should assume substantial responsibility for their own health brought a new dimension to the management of health care services and opened up for the Member States of WHO an opportunity to redraft and expand their health services. At the Alma-Ata Conference, organized jointly by WHO and UNICEF in 1978, 137 States unanimously accepted the primary health care approach as the most effective way of achieving health for all by the year 2000.

Part 1 of this publication is a working guide intended for use by community health workers in developing countries as a learning text and as a guide in their work. It outlines the structure and content of the CHW's training on the basis of the most common aspects of their work. The following criteria have been applied in the selection of training topics:

—demand from the public;
—frequency of the disease or condition;
—danger to the community;
—danger to the individual;
—technical feasibility of action for a CHW;
—economic consequences of the disease or condition.

Part 2 is addressed to the teachers, tutors, and supervisors of CHWs. Part 3 discusses the adaptation of the book to local conditions, which can be undertaken only in the country where it is to be used.

This publication is not specific to any one country and must be *adapted* to local needs, structures, and potentialities.

The community health worker (CHW) profile

What is a CHW?

CHWs are men and women chosen by the community, and trained to deal with the health problems of individuals and the community, and to work in close relationship with the health services.

They should have had a level of primary education that enables them to read, write and do simple mathematical calculations.

Conditions of work

CHWs are responsible both to local community authorities and to supervisors appointed by the health services. They are expected to follow their supervisor's guidance in a health team relationship.

CHWs, who may be employed full-time or part-time in health work, are paid in money or in kind by the local community or by the health services.

Generally, the local community provides a house or room and basic equipment, to be used only for health work.

What do community health workers do?

As already noted, this publication is not specific to any one country, and consequently does not provide a job description for CHWs; this will vary from one place to another. However, as examples, the table on page 12 lists the major tasks that CHWs are expected to perform in 11 countries (see also Unit 49, "Knowing your work clearly").

Their duties will cover both health care and community development, but what they do should be restricted to what they have learned in training. They must recognize their limitations and work within those limitations. They cannot be expected to solve all the problems they meet, but they should be able to deal with those that are the most common and urgent.

CHWs should always bear in mind that they are not working in isolation. Rather, they function within a health system and should be guided and supported by skilled supervisors. They should know where and when to seek guidance, and refer or seek help for patients who are seriously ill or whose treatment is beyond their competence. Many times in this guide, the CHW is instructed to obtain a supervisor's advice or to send the patient to the health centre or hospital; this clearly indicates that CHWs cannot and should not try to do everything alone. It can never be emphasized enough that the quality of the services provided by CHWs depends on the skill and dedication of each individual CHW, the quality of their training, skilled and supportive supervision, a reliable communication network (postal and telephone services, transport etc.), and a reliable referral system linking the CHW to a health centre or a first-level hospital.

Duties of community health workers in different countries

TASK SUMMARY	BENIN	BOTSWANA	COLOMBIA	INDIA	JAMAICA	LIBERIA	PAPUA NEW GUINEA	PHILIP-PINES	SUDAN	THAILAND	YEMEN
1 First aid, treat accident and simple illness	/	/	/	/	/	/	/	/	/	/	/
2 Dispense drugs	/	/	(including injections)	/	/	/	(including injections)	/	/	(VHV only)	/
3 Pre- and post-natal advice, motivation	/	/	/	/	/	/	/	/	/	/	/
4 Deliver babies	/	X	/	X	X	X	X	X	X	X	X
5 Child-care advice, motivation	/	/	/	/	/	/	/	/	/	/	/
6 Nutrition motivation, demonstration	/	/	/	/	/	/	/	/	/	/	/
7 Nutrition action (W = weigh children, maintain chart; F = distribute food supplements)	F	W	W	X	W, F	X	W	W, F	F	W, F	X
8 Immunization motivation, assistance during clinic	/	/	/	/	/	/	/	/	/	/	/
9 Immunization—give injections	X	X	/	X	X	X	/	X	/	X	X
10 Family planning motivation	/	/	/	/	/	/	X	/	/	/	/
11 Family planning—distribute supplies	X	/	/	/	X	X	X	/	/	/	X
12 Environmental sanitation, personal hygiene, general health habits—motivation	/	/	/	/	/	/	/	/	/	/	/
13 Communicable disease screening, referral, prevention, motivation	/	/	/	/	X	/	/	/	/	/	/
14 Communicable disease follow-up, motivation of confirmed cases	/	/	/	/	X	sometimes	/	/	/	/	sometimes
15 Communicable disease action (D = provide drug resupply; M = take malaria slide)	X	D	D, M	M	X	X	D, M	TB sputum smear	D	X	D
16 Assist health centre clinic activities (i.e., not in village)	occasion-ally	/	occasion-ally	X	/	X	/	X	occasion-ally	X	X
17 Refer difficult cases to health centre or hospital	/	/	/	/	/	/	/	/	/	/	/
18 Perform school health activities regularly	X	/	X	X	X	X	X	X	/	X	/
19 Collect vital statistics	X	/	/	/	X	/	X	/	/	/	/
20 Maintain records, reports	/	/	/	/	/	/	/	/	/	/	/
21 Visit homes on a regular basis	/	/	/	/	/	sometimes	/	/	/	(VHV only)	/
22 Perform tasks outside health sector (e.g., agriculture)	/	/	X	/	X	/	X	/	/	/	X
23 Participate in community meetings	/	/	/	/	/	/	/	/	/	/	/

KEY: / = task not performed by CHW   X = task performed by CHW

Source: Community health workers, unpublished WHO document, SHS/HMD/84.1, 1984.

CHWs should help local authorities and the public to take initiatives and should show an interest in any activity likely to improve the people's living conditions. They should always consider what can be done locally with the community's own resources, and at the least possible cost. They should always remember that health cannot be the responsibility of the health sector alone, and that important contributions to people's health are made by many other sectors, such as education, agriculture, public works, and communications.

What training will CHWs receive?

This will depend on their job description, the problems they have to solve, the level of development of the country or area, and their previous education.

For CHWs working in rural areas in a developing country, the initial training may be for as little as six to eight weeks, but it can be longer. The training must be practical and should preferably be given in the health service area where they live and will work. As far as possible, supervisors should play an important part in the training. Supervision should also include continuing, on-the-spot training as well as provision for refresher courses and training for new skills at the health centre or elsewhere. A plan for this further training should be worked out.

Part 1

Working Guide

> **_Bear in mind that:_**
>
> ■ _Several community health workers (CHWs) may work as a team in the same village with their supervisors_
>
> ■ _Certain health tasks may be tackled best by a male CHW and others by a female CHW, depending on the wishes of the community, its customs and its resources_
>
> ■ _A CHW does not work in isolation. He should be a part of the health system and should be regularly supervised. He should know when and how to seek guidance and to refer patients who are seriously ill to a doctor for treatment._

Chapter 1
Knowing your community

Unit 1
Learning about the community

A community is made up of many kinds of people. If you understand how they organize themselves for various purposes, it will be easier for you to help them to be healthy.

To be healthy, people must eat enough good food, drink clean water, work and live in a clean environment, and have healthy habits.

To improve life in a community you must know who is healthy and who is not, and why these people are not healthy.

Learning objectives

After studying this unit you should be able to:

1 Find out the number of people, families, and households that make up the community.

2 Find out who are the people who make important decisions about the community or who have influence over decisions about the community.

3 Find out, by talking with the community leaders, what are the main problems, concerns, and causes of bad health in your community.

4 Draw, with the help of the schoolteacher and others, a map of your area showing where people live and the main landmarks, such as groups of houses, main buildings, rivers, wells, and ponds.

5 Help the community to decide what it wants to improve first and how to get it done.

How many people, families, and households are there in the community?

To help people to be healthy, you must know your community very well. You must count how many people there are in the community, and how many of them are young, middle-aged, and old. You should also know: who are the very poor people who cannot buy enough food to stay healthy; which households have latrines and which do not; and which households have a water supply or a private well and which do not.

Who are the leaders in your community?

Find out who makes the decisions for the community. These people are the leaders. They may be tribal leaders, religious leaders, or political leaders. It is usually the leaders who can best help you to do your work well.

There are often other people whose opinions and decisions are valued, such as the elderly, land-owners, money-lenders, or businessmen. You will need to know who these people are and how to get their support for your work.

Find out how the community is organized and who runs its affairs. For example:

■ Which group makes decisions for all the people? Is it a development committee, a party committee, or some other group?

■ Does this group deal with all the affairs of the community? Or does it form subcommittees that look after different needs of the community, e.g., health, water supply, and education?

■ Is there a health committee? Who are its members? Are they appointed or elected? What are their tasks? How often do they meet? Who calls them together? Are all sections or groups in the community represented?

■ What other groups are there? For example, a women's group or a farmers' cooperative.

Try to get to know the village or community groups well so that you can get their support for your health work.

What are the main health problems and what are their causes?

You may already know many things about your community when you begin your health work, especially if it is a small community. You will learn more by talking with leaders and other people. Some of the common causes of bad health are:

■ there are too many people living close together

■ there is not enough water or the water is not clean

■ there is not enough food of the right kind

■ there are unclean houses in dirty surroundings

■ there is no way to keep cool in the heat or to keep warm in the cold

■ there are no or too few latrines or the latrines are dirty

■ the people do not protect themselves from insects that carry diseases

■ the people cannot get to the health centre easily

■ their working conditions are unhealthy

■ the people cannot read and thus do not learn about health and healthy habits.

What are the main concerns of the people?

You should visit and talk with various groups and people: families or households (both rich and poor), those who make decisions for the community about the community, members of special groups. Try to find out:

■ what part of their available resources do they devote to health?

■ what community problems are they especially concerned about?

■ what have they been doing about these problems?

■ what do they think can be done?

- how would they like you to help them in solving these problems?

If you can help the people in solving or reducing these problems you will be improving their health. However, quite often, you may find that what people think their health problems are, or what they think the causes of sickness are, are different from what the staff of the health centre think. You may also find that people do not often connect their health problems with other common problems such as a bad water supply, poor communications, or scarcity of fuel.

If, for example, the problems of the community are concerned with water supply, communications, and fuel you will need to ask questions such as:

(1) *Water supply*. What are the different ways in which people get water for drinking, bathing, watering animals, and watering crops and gardens. Is the water safe to drink or wash with? Does it cause sickness? Is water available throughout the year?

(2) *Transport and communications*. How do people go to markets, schools, health centres, hospitals? How can messages be sent to other places, to health centres? How can you receive messages from other places, from your supervisor?

(3) *Fuel*. What do the people use for cooking and heating (electricity, kerosene, wood, gas, coal, cow-dung), and for light? Is it too expensive for poor families? Can households boil their water easily? Can they cook their food properly?

All the above questions affect health and disease. As a community health worker you will need to make the people aware of these problems as part of their education for improving health.

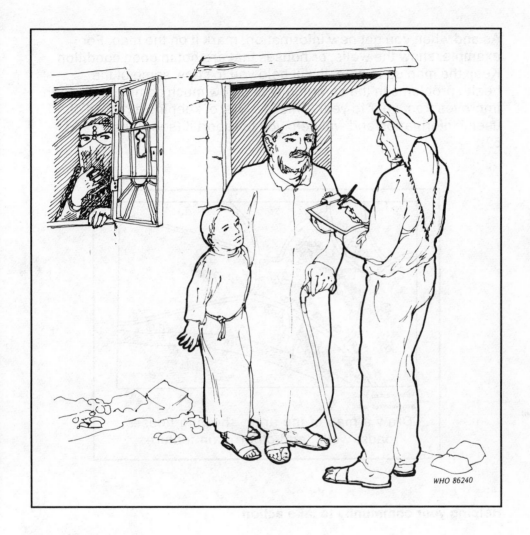

WHO 86240

Drawing a map of your area

If there is not already a good map of your area and the village, ask some people (for example, the schoolteacher and schoolchildren) to help you to draw one. Ask them to show the rivers, parks, schools, temples, roads and other important places. For a small community, the map can show all the houses in the area. Take the map to the community committee and place it where the people can see it.

As and when you get new information, mark it on the map. For example, show the wells, or houses that are not in good condition. Keep the map up to date. It will help you to show some of the health problems in the community and how much community health improves from year to year. This is a way of keeping a record of useful information and will help you to report it (see Units 51 and 52).

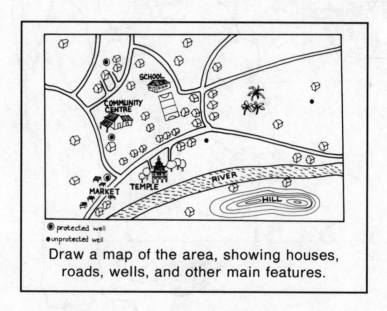

● protected well
● unprotected well

Draw a map of the area, showing houses, roads, wells, and other main features.

Helping your community to take action

You must have the support of your community committee and other groups.

The community committee and the people do not think about health problems separately from other problems. They think about the land, crops, food, water, housing, etc. together. You must be concerned about the general well-being of the people and not simply about their illnesses. Your task is to help them to understand that they must take certain actions themselves to keep in good health.

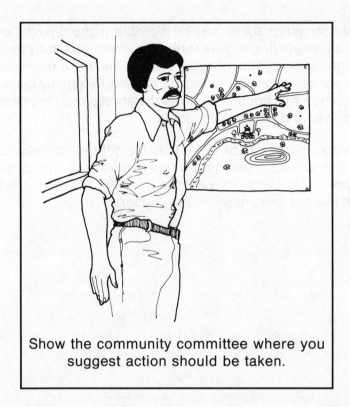

Show the community committee where you
suggest action should be taken.

Find out what the committee thinks are the most important
problems of the people, and what resources the community has to
solve them.

Find out what the committee thinks can be done about the
problems. Then see what you can do to help.

Always discuss with the community leaders and the people what
you think should be done to make life better. For example, the
committee may decide that the village must be cleaned up. Your
task will be to discuss with the committee:

- how to form cleaning teams, what their tasks should be, and how
  to use them

- when and where to start

- when to report back on progress made.

On another occasion, there may be a problem about young children being left alone playing in the street. The committee may ask the women's group or a youth group to help in making a playground or a day-care centre for the children. You could help by discussing with the women's or youth group which of these two proposals will be appropriate and how to carry it out.

Usually, many things can be done to solve different problems, but you will have to help in deciding which of the various proposals is the best one to start with. Remember, this should be the one that most people want and are willing to support.

Unit 2

Epidemics

When several people have the same sickness at about the same time, this is an epidemic. An epidemic happens when a sickness passes from one person to others in a group, such as children at school or people in a community, or when several people eat the same contaminated food.

Learning objectives

After studying this unit you should be able to:

1 Explain to the people what an epidemic is and how it happens.

2 Describe to them how you and the community can prevent epidemics from starting.

3 Describe also how you and the community can prevent epidemics from spreading.

How does an epidemic happen?

An epidemic happens when many people have a disease, such as a cold, a cough, or diarrhoea and vomiting, at the same time. There can be an epidemic of measles or whooping cough among the children of a community where the babies or young children have not been immunized against these diseases.

When only a few children get tuberculosis at about the same time, this is a small epidemic; it usually means that the children have got the disease from the same person or perhaps from drinking the milk of a cow that has tuberculosis.

Sometimes an epidemic happens suddenly, for example, when families or other groups eat bad food that carries germs or drink dirty water or a poisonous liquor at a marriage or festival, and all get sick at the same time.

Usually, a coughing sickness with fever starts with a few people and then spreads quickly from one person to another, until many people in the community have it at the same time. Most people get better without treatment, but some weak or badly nourished young children or old people may die from the sickness.

How to prevent epidemics from starting

Make sure that:

- All the babies and children in the community are immunized against the six diseases mentioned in Unit 21. This will prevent epidemics of tuberculosis, diphtheria, whooping cough, tetanus, poliomyelitis and measles.

- All babies are breast-fed. This will protect them from diarrhoea caused by dirty food and water. Breast milk also protects children from coughing diseases.

- The food and water in a community are safe. This avoids epidemics of diarrhoea and vomiting.

- Latrines are built and used properly. This helps prevent epidemics of diarrhoea and intestinal worms.

You should also discuss with parents, children, and community groups how epidemics can be prevented.

How can you help prevent epidemics from spreading?

As soon as you find out that there is an epidemic in your community, you should:

- Inform your supervisor, the community leaders, and the school-teachers, that an epidemic has started.

- Advise people who are sick not to come close to other people.

- Advise families to keep their babies, young children and elderly away from sick people and from places where people gather together.

- Treat patients who have:
  fever (see Unit 24)
  cough (see Unit 25)
  diarrhoea (see Unit 26)
  intestinal worms (see Unit 38).

When you find whole familes or groups becoming sick suddenly with diarrhoea, vomiting and belly pains, this is usually because all have eaten the same bad food or drunk bad water or another drink at the same time from one place. You should inform the health centre at once and ask your supervisor for help. Try to find out where the bad food and drink came from, or whether all the sick people had taken water from the same well. If a certain food or drink is found to be the cause of this sickness, then the community leaders should inform people that no one should take this bad food or bad drink again until your supervisor or the doctor from the health centre says it is safe to do so (see Units 5 and 26).

> ### *Always take advantage of an epidemic:*
>
> - *To discuss the problem with the community leaders and families*
>
> - *To encourage them to decide what they can do to prevent it from happening again*
>
> - *To remind people that many epidemics can be prevented by immunization, keeping food and water clean, controlling the insects and animals that carry disease, and by regularly taking the medicine that prevents malaria.*

Chapter 2
Promoting a healthy environment in the community

Unit 3
Housing

The house is the centre of family life. The kinds of houses in which people live affect their health. Good houses protect health. Bad houses may damage health.

The CHW should know how housing affects health and should be able to advise people on how to improve their houses in order to have a healthier environment and better health.

In judging how good a house is, consider five important points:

- *the site of the house*

- *the amount of space, the layout, and the ventilation*

- *protection against rain and wind, heat and cold, insects and animals*

- *materials used in constructing the house*

- *how people maintain and use their house.*

Learning objectives

After studying this unit you should be able to:

1 Give advice on where to site a house.

2 Give advice on space, layout, and ventilation of a house.

3 Explain to the people what is needed for a house to give the necessary protection.

4 Explain to them how floors and walls may be made safe.

5 Explain the need to clean and maintain the house, and warn against overcrowding.

A healthy house

A healthy house need not be a big house made of modern materials. Traditional houses often suit people's needs and activities and the local climate better than "modern" houses. Often, traditional houses can be made more healthy if attention is paid to cleanliness and simple improvements that do not cost much.

You should speak to your supervisor about how housing can best be improved in your area. He can tell you what to look for to see whether a house is healthy, and how to improve it in the easiest and cheapest way.

The site of the house

The site of the house is important for health. For example, a house should not be sited close to a place where people dump waste. This is because there will be many flies, other insects, and rats near the waste dump and these animals spread disease. If rainwater floods the site, or if groundwater seeps into the walls, the house will be damp and unhealthy.

The exposure of the site to the sun should be considered: in a cool or cold climate the sun can heat the walls; in a hot climate the site should be shaded from the sun as much as possible, for example by choosing a site which is surrounded by trees.

In general, a healthy house is:

- close to a reliable supply of safe water (see Unit 4);
- more than 100 metres away from a place where people dump waste (see Unit 6);
- close to a sanitary means of disposal of excreta (see Unit 7);
- in a place from which rainwater and waste water drain away and where puddles do not form.

Space, layout and ventilation of a house

Space

When a house is very crowded, diseases spread more easily from person to person. More space is better for health.

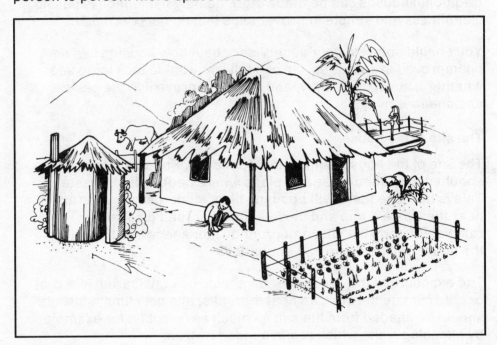

Layout

Waste water and waste are full of germs that may cause disease. There must be a way of draining away waste water, or of using it to water a garden. Solid waste should be disposed of safely because waste attracts flies and other insects and animals which may spread disease.

Domestic animals should be kept in a separate area so as to avoid bringing dirt into the house where people live. A fence should keep out hens, goats and other animals.

Every house should have a latrine of its own (see Unit 7).

The house should be safe for young children. Anything that might hurt them, such as fire, knives, medicines, or chemicals used in the garden, should be kept out of their reach. Small children should not be allowed in the cooking area.

Ventilation

It is important to have fresh air blowing freely through the house so that smoke and stale air clear quickly. This can be done by positioning doors and windows in such a way that air can pass freely through the rooms of the house. If the windows have to be kept shut in the cold season, then the house should have a chimney or a hole in the roof to let out the smoke from the fire.

In general, a healthy house has:

- enough space so that people are not crowded together, especially when sleeping
- barriers to keep animals out and a fenced-off area, at least 10 m from the house and from outdoor living areas, for goats, sheep, pigs, cows, or other domestic animals
- separate places for bathing and washing household utensils and clothes, with drainage of waste water to plants in the garden
- a place to store food and water, which can be reached easily but can also be kept very clean and safe from rats, mice and other animals and insects (see Unit 5)
- a place for a fire or cooking stove (under a chimney or an opening in the roof to let out the smoke), which is protected to minimize danger of burns and scalds, especially to little children
- windows that permit cross-currents of air so that fresh air may enter and stale or smoky air may be drawn or blown out
- protected places to store dangerous substances and objects out of the reach of children.

A house should provide the necessary protection

A healthy house is neither too warm nor too cold—people should feel comfortable in it.

There should be a door to keep animals out. Food in the house should be stored in such a way that rats and mice cannot reach it.

If possible, doors and windows should have net screens to keep flies and mosquitos out. Mosquito nets can also be used over beds while people are sleeping.

In warm climates, the walls should be protected from the sun by, for example, sunshades or a simple veranda, around the house.

Rainwater should flow from the roof into a gutter that leads into a drain or container; this keeps the walls and the ground around the house dry.

In general, a healthy house has:

- a good roof to keep out the rain
- good walls and doors to protect against bad weather, and to keep out animals
- screens of netting wire at the windows and doors to keep out insects, especially mosquitos
- sunshades all around to protect the walls from direct sunlight in hot weather.

Floors and walls should be made safe

Always remember that local materials and local constructions can often be very good and healthy. Bricks, cement, and corrugated iron sheets are not necessarily better than traditional materials which have always served their purpose well. The so-called "modern" ways of building houses are not always better than the old ways.

Whenever possible, building materials that do not burn easily should be chosen instead of materials that catch fire easily.

In general, a healthy house has:

- a floor of wood, stamped clay, bamboo, concrete, tiles, or similar material so that people do not have to walk on the bare earth and so that the floor can be easily cleaned;

- walls with a smooth hard surface so that they can be easily cleaned and with no holes or cracks in which insects, rodents or other carriers of disease can live.

A house should be clean, well maintained and not overcrowded

The way people use their house can affect their health. Every house, no matter how small or what materials it is made of, can be made more healthy by regular cleaning, removal of refuse, timely repairs, and conscientious use of latrines (see Unit 7). When too many people live in one house, it makes cleaning and maintenance difficult, causes tension among the occupants, and may result in respiratory infections.

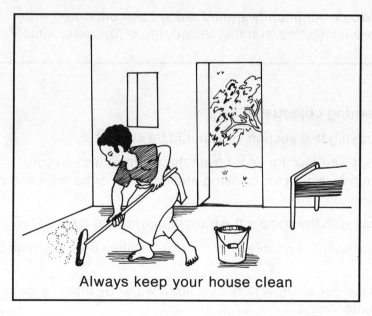

Always keep your house clean

Unit 4
Water supply

Much sickness is caused by dirty or unsafe water.

To be healthy, people need clean water for:

- *drinking*
- *preparing and cooking food*
- *washing the body*
- *washing clothes.*

A clean water supply is essential for community health. Clean water comes from a protected tap, spring, well, or borehole. Water for drinking from any other source should first be treated to make it safe. When it cannot be boiled, it should be cleaned by filtration. The vessels and other containers used for storing or carrying water must be kept clean.

The whole community should always be concerned with improving and maintaining the quality of the water supply.

Learning objectives

After studying this section you should be able to:

1 Find out whether the water from the water source in your community is safe for drinking and cooking, or bathing and other uses.

2 Discuss with the people the danger of drinking dirty water.

3 Discuss with the people how they can protect their sources of water.

4 Show the people how they can clean water by filtering, boiling or disinfecting it.

5 Discuss with the people why they should keep clean and cover carefully the vessels and tanks in which they store water.

Dirty water causes diarrhoea

If people often get diarrhoea in your community you should check where people get their water from and how they use it. The use of unclean water is often a main cause of diarrhoea.

Visit the places where the people get their water from and decide what is wrong and what action should be taken to improve the situation.

The people usually get water from:

- a pond
- a river
- a spring
- a well or a borehole
- a tank (rainwater).

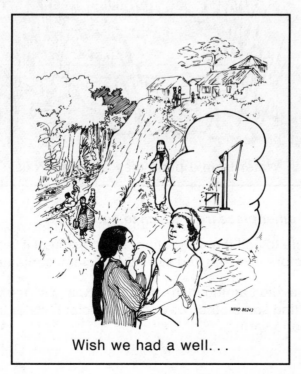

Wish we had a well. . .

The people may be drawing the water directly from the source or the water may be coming through pipes to a common village tap or stand-pipe or to separate house connections.

Watch how they draw their drinking-water from the source and how they carry and store it. Visit houses to find out what they do to keep their drinking-water clean.

Water from a pond

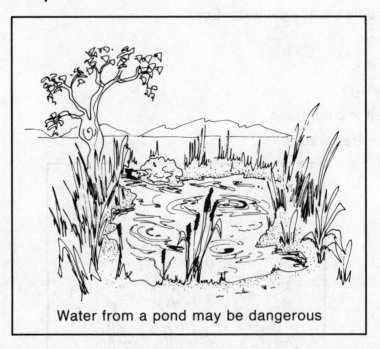

Water from a pond may be dangerous

If there is no other place from which to get water

Tell the people to boil the water, filter it, or disinfect it with chemicals before drinking and store it in a clean container.

They should avoid bathing in the pond. Discuss with the village chief how to find some other way of getting clean water such as from a river or a spring.

If there is another place (river, spring or well) from which to get water

First make sure the other sources are clean and not too far away. Then advise the people not to use water from the pond for drinking.

The pond can then be used for other purposes such as watering the cattle, or watering gardens, but not for drinking or cooking.

Water from a river

If there is no other place to get water from

The people should draw water from the river before it reaches the village (see drawing below, point no. 1) and boil, filter, or disinfect the water before drinking it.

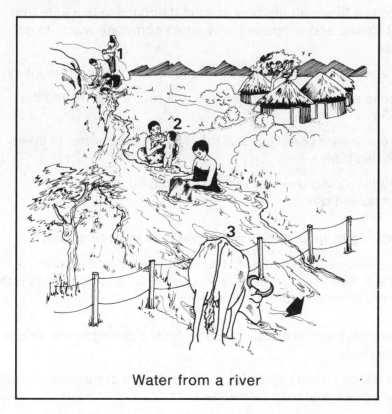

Water from a river

They should bathe and wash clothes only where the river leaves the village, and only let the animals drink the water further down the river (see drawing, page 39, points 2 and 3).

Ask your supervisor if it is safe for people to bathe in the river.

If there is a well or a spring

Advise the people that it is safer to get drinking-water from a well or spring if the water from these sources is known to be clean. See the next two sections on wells and springs.

Water from a spring

Spring water is usually clean, but only if the spring is well protected. A spring is properly protected when

■ there is a fence all the way around it and there is a gate that is kept closed and is opened only when someone wants to get water;

■ there is a ditch around the spring to let the water drain away

■ there is a cemented stone wall half a metre high round the spring

■ there is a pipe coming out of this wall and the water is taken from this pipe

■ there is a cover over the spring to keep out animals, birds, insects, and dirt.

If the spring is not properly protected or is not being used

See the village chief and help the village to have it properly protected. See your supervisor if you cannot arrange to get water from the spring or protect it properly.

If the people want to bring the water from a spring to the village through pipes

This is usually a very good idea. Consult your supervisor about any help or advice that may be needed.

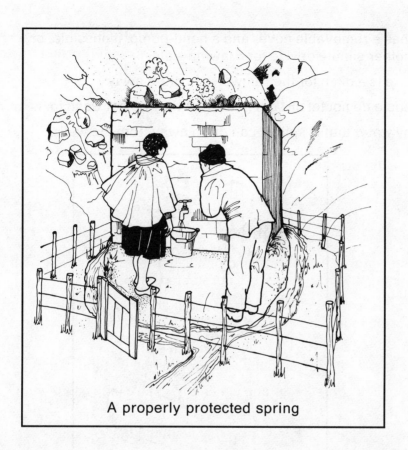

A properly protected spring

Water from a well

Water from a well is usually clean, but only if the well is properly protected.

A well is properly protected if:

- it is at least 20 metres away and uphill from any latrine or rubbish heap

- it is at least 3 metres deep

- it is lined inside with stones stuck with mortar

- there is a stone wall around it which is at least half a metre high

- it has a removable cover and a hand-pump, if possible, or another simple device for drawing water
- there is a ditch for the rainwater to drain away
- people do not let dirt get into it and they do not wash in it
- any water that is spilled can drain away from the well.

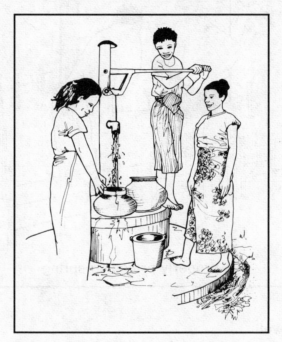

If the well is not protected

Discuss with the community committee how the well may be protected. Talk with your supervisor about choosing a place for a new well if necessary.

If the people want to improve the well (by putting in a pump, for example) or if they are talking about drilling to search for water, ask your supervisor's advice.

Water from a rainwater tank

If rainwater is collected in tanks for drinking and cooking, explain to the people how to keep the tank-water clean.

The water in the tank will be clean if:

- it enters the tank through a screen or a filter to keep out leaves, dirt, and insects
- the tank is covered to keep out dirt and insects
- the tank is emptied and cleaned at the beginning of the rainy season
- the water is taken from the tank either through a tap (above-ground tank), or with a hand-pump or a hand-winch (below-ground tank).

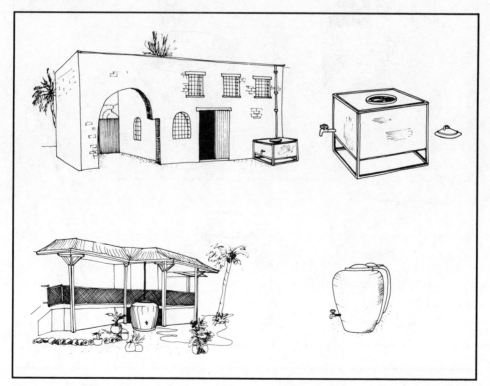

People carry water from the well or spring in a container and store it at home

The water can be kept clean if the container:

■ is kept clean

■ is cleaned and rinsed before it is filled

■ is disinfected with bleaching powder (see Annex 2) or by boiling water in it

■ is used only for clean water

■ is kept covered with a clean cloth or lid.

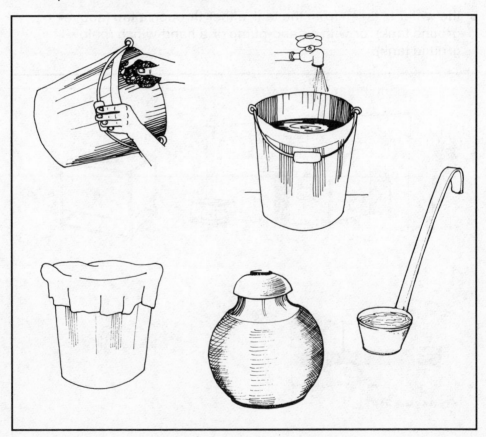

Do not put hands or dirty cups or dippers into the water. Use a clean cup with a long handle to take water out.

Filtration of water

Filtering water does not disinfect it, as boiling does, but it is a simple way of removing some disease-causing germs and eggs of some worms. Filtering will make the water less dangerous.

Instructions on how to make a filter are given in Annex 2.

Chlorination of water

It is possible to purify water and make it safe for drinking by adding to it a disinfectant such as chlorine.

Chlorination of water is a procedure that is best implemented at the community level. Ask your supervisor for advice. A chlorination technique using bleaching powder is described in Annex 2.

Unit 5
Food safety

Food is very precious. People should not let it go bad or be eaten or spoiled by rats and other animals.

It should be kept clean at every stage — from production until it is eaten. Stale or contaminated food can cause diarrhoea and other diseases.

Food can also be contaminated by chemicals through:

- *careless use of household insecticides*
- *careless use of pesticides by the farmer*
- *treatment of seeds with chemicals*
- *accidental contamination during transport and storage.*

You should know how to prevent the diseases or sicknesses that people can get from eating stale or contaminated foods.

Learning objectives

After studying this unit you should be able to:

1 Find out what the people in your community eat, and how they prepare and store food.

2 Explain to them how food animals should be hygienically slaughtered and offered for sale.

3 Discuss with the community leaders, families and those who handle or sell food the risks to health of eating contaminated food and how to prevent contamination of food.

4 Explain to the people how to store food and how to protect it from rodents, insects, flies, and dirt.

Contaminated food can cause diarrhoea

If there are 5 or more new patients with diarrhoea in 1 week, or your supervisor has asked you what you have done since his last visit to have the village food protected, or you have noticed that food is stored carelessly or that meat or fish is put on sale from dirty stalls in the market, or the pond from which fish come is polluted, what are you going to do?

Find out:

- what the people eat
- how they prepare their food
- how they store their food.

Then decide what action to take.

What do the people eat?

Grain (wheat, rice, millet or other)

The main problems with grain concern storage. See section on storage on page 51.

Vegetables

Vegetables that will be eaten raw should not be fertilized with faeces. When faeces have been used as fertilizer, vegetables should always be well washed and properly cooked before they are eaten.

Meat

Eating raw or undercooked meat can be very dangerous. Eating infected or contaminated meat can cause severe vomiting and diarrhoea, infestation with worms, and other illnesses that sometimes cause death.

Food animals should be slaughtered hygienically and in a way that prevents disease. The food animals should be healthy. They should be hanging during slaughter, and after that they should be fully bled. The slaughterhouse (abattoir) or the place of slaughtering should be fenced off and kept clean. Diseased parts (e.g., liver with worms) found during removal of the offal and processing of the carcass should be burned or buried and *not* given to dogs.

Meat shops should be kept clean. Meat should be sold separately from other foods, in special covered shops. A large cut of meat should be kept hanging before it is sold, and it should be protected from insects and animals. The butcher should wash his hands very well before he begins the sale of the meat. He should also wash his hands with soap each time he goes to the lavatory (latrine), and should use a clean cloth to dry his hands. The butcher should make sure that all cutting instruments and the surfaces on which meat is cut are kept clean.

Advise the butcher on how to keep the shop and meat clean. Visit the shop from time to time to make sure he is following your advice. If you find that he is not following your advice, inform the community committee and other leaders.

Handling meat in the house. Surfaces on which meat is cut and instruments used for cutting raw meat should be very well washed and dried before use. Utensils in which meat is cooked and served should also be cleaned in a similar way. To prevent spoilage, meat may be dried, or salted, or cooked immediately. Properly dried and salted meat will keep for a long time. Cooked meat should be eaten at once or within a very short time of cooking.

Fish

Fish is a very good food, but it can go bad very quickly in warm climates, sometimes even within a few hours of being caught. Fish and shellfish can spread many diseases caused by germs and poisons, especially if it has been caught in polluted water or if it is eaten raw or undercooked.

Fresh fish should always be:

- gutted as soon as possible
- kept away from direct sunlight and dry wind

- kept as cold as possible

- cooked and eaten without delay.

If fish is not to be eaten very soon it may be cured (that is, salted, smoked, or dried).

If the water (sea, lake, river, pond) in which the fish or shellfish is caught is polluted with sewage, faeces, or animal waste, the fish should not be eaten raw. If the water is polluted with discharge from factories or with oil, the fish will often be dangerous to eat. You should discuss this problem with the community committee and ask your supervisor for help in dealing with it.

Milk

Milk is a very good food, but it can pass on several diseases from the cow, camel, or goat to the person who drinks it. It can also become contaminated by dirt from the animal and from the hands or throat (through coughing) of the milk handler, and in that way spread disease.

If milk has to be stored for use during the day, boil it every 4–5 hours. If it has to be left overnight, boil it and keep it in a cool place away from insects, rodents, and cats. Boil the milk again in the morning before use.

To avoid diseases spread by milk:

- take the milk only from healthy-looking animals

- wash the animal's udder before milking; the milker's hands should also be washed

- boil the milk before drinking it

- store milk in clean vessels in which water has been boiled or which have been rinsed with hot water.

Eggs

Eggs provide essential body-building food. Hens' eggs may be eaten raw when fresh. Duck eggs should always be cooked.

Fruit

Fresh fruit contains vitamins and minerals, which are very good for the body. Fruit should be eaten fresh after being washed or peeled.

How to prevent contamination of food

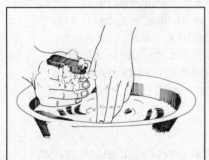

People who handle, prepare, and serve food should wash their hands well, with clean water and soap. They should always keep any finger wounds bandaged cleanly. The tables or other surfaces on which food is prepared, and the utensils used, should be kept clean.

Show the women who prepare food at home how to wash and dry their hands properly and to clean their nails.

Show the people who work in the restaurants and food shops how to wash and dry their hands properly. Ask the village chief to remind the people in the community from time to time to wash their hands before they touch food, especially after they have been to the latrine.

People should also be reminded regularly to:

- cook food for only one meal at a time, unless they can chill the leftovers
- see that the food is eaten soon after it is cooked—food should not be left for long in a warm place.

How should people store their food?

Storing cooked food

Put the food in a clean container in which water has just been boiled or which has been rinsed with hot water. Cover the container with a clean cloth. Store it in a cool place which is protected against flies, other insects, mice, rats, and other animals.

In hot countries, people often store drinking-water in a shaded, but breezy, corner of the house. This keeps the water cool. It is a good idea to store cooked food near the drinking-water vessel. This will keep the food cool and unspoiled for a few hours. If earthen pots are used to store water, the place around the vessel will be even cooler.

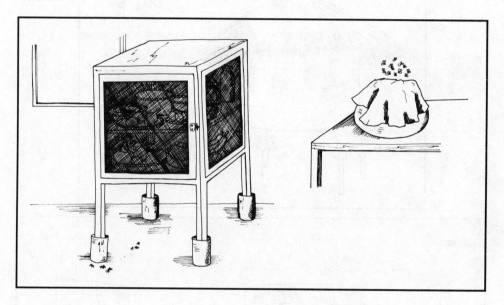

Storage of grain

The grain store is properly protected against rats if:

- it is closed on all sides
- it is raised at least 30 cm above the ground
- there is no grain (or other food) lying around near it or near the house
- there is a lid to close the container properly
- metallic cones are placed on the poles that support the container to prevent the rats from climbing up

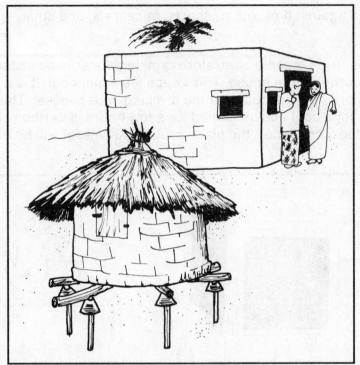

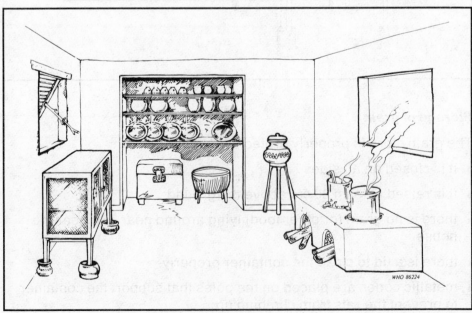

If you see a grain store that is not properly protected against rats, show the head of the household what to do (see page 51). If after a month there are still some rats, consult your supervisor.

Always remember!

Dirty food brings disease (particularly diarrhoea) to the whole family

To avoid wasting food:

- *prevent flies, worms, rats and other animals from reaching the food and eating or contaminating it*

- *eat the food soon after it is cooked.*

To keep the food clean and safe:

- *wash your hands before touching or preparing food*

- *prevent dust from the house and the road, flies, clothes, mice, rats, animals, and children's or adults' hands from touching what is going to be eaten*

- *cook enough food for one meal only and never keep left-overs if you cannot chill them*

- *keep your kitchen utensils clean*

- *do not leave clean utensils lying on the ground.*

Unit 6

Getting rid of waste

Every household produces waste (or rubbish) from cooking, eating, sweeping, cleaning, and other work. If this rubbish is left lying around the house it becomes dangerous. In hot climates it should be removed daily.

To stay healthy, a household must get rid of its waste safely.

Learning objectives

After studying this unit you should be able to:

1 Tell the people which main health problems are caused by unsafe ways of getting rid of waste.

2 Find out how families get rid of their household waste.

3 Discuss with them whether what they do is safe and how to make it safer.

4 Propose to the village chief or committee what might be done by the whole community and by individual households to get rid of household waste properly.

Main health problems caused by waste

When waste is left lying around it makes the area look dirty and it produces a bad smell. It also attracts flies and rats and other animals which can carry disease germs to the people. For example, if flies that have been sitting on dirty waste sit on food, the people who eat the food can become ill.

If waste is left to rot near a river, pond, well or spring there is the danger that it will come into contact with the drinking-water and make it dirty. When people drink this dirty water they can get diarrhoea and other diseases.

If children get hurt when playing with waste or near it, their wounds can become badly infected.

Therefore, **waste must never be left lying around**. It should be got rid of safely. Find out where people throw their waste, discuss with them what they do, and suggest what action to take.

Dumping waste in a common pit

In most villages there is a common pit where people throw their waste. This pit should be properly protected from animals and flies in order to prevent diseases in the community. A common pit is properly placed and protected if:

- it is outside the village and at least 20 metres away from the nearest house
- it is in a hollow and not on a hill
- it is at least 100 metres away from any river, well or spring
- there is a fence around it
- the waste is piled up in a hole and not scattered around
- the waste is kept covered with earth at least 2 or 3 cm deep
- surface water cannot run into it.

If the pit is not being properly used, discuss with the chief how the village can have a good common pit. Once proper arrangements are made, see whether it is being properly used by visiting it regularly.

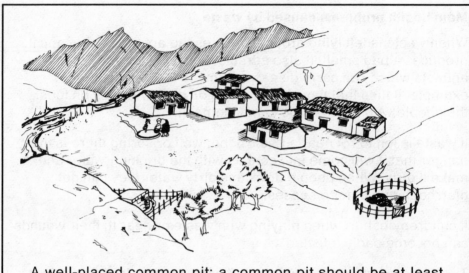

A well-placed common pit: a common pit should be at least
20 metres from the nearest house and 100 metres from any river,
well or spring

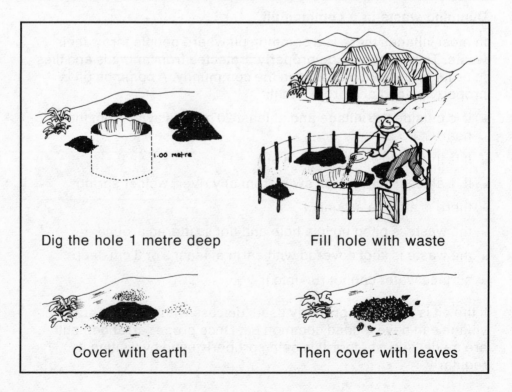

Dig the hole 1 metre deep

Fill hole with waste

Cover with earth

Then cover with leaves

When there is no common pit

(1) If people throw waste around their house, this can be dangerous. People can get diarrhoea and other diseases if the waste is left rotting around the house. You should discuss this matter with the people and the village chief, and try to get a common pit ready as soon as possible. Make sure that the common pit is safe and well protected (see previous sections on

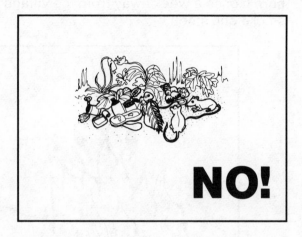

dumping of waste in a common pit). It will be useful to ask your supervisor to come and advise on how to dig a pit or on other ways of disposing of and burning waste.

(2) If people throw waste near a river, well or spring or near a drain that flows into the river, there is a danger that the water may become dirty. If people drink such dirty water they may become ill. Discuss this problem with the

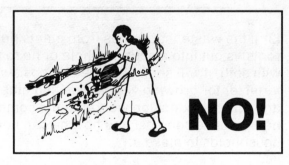

village chief and your supervisor. Try to get a common pit dug. Make sure it is used properly.

Other suggestions you can make for getting rid of waste

(1) Bury the waste in a hole at a safe distance from the houses and from sources of drinking-water.

(2) Collect the waste in a container or make a neat heap of it and burn it once a week away from the village to avoid problems of smoke and smell.

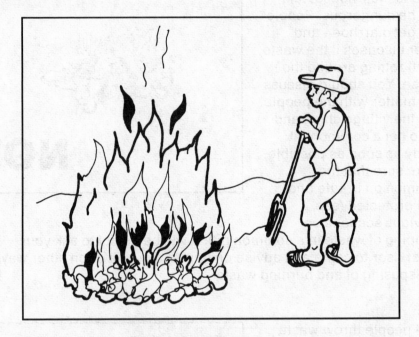

(3) If the waste that comes from plants (leaves, vegetables, fruit, roots) is put into a separate hole or heap (and if possible mixed with soil), it will soon become compost, which can be used as fertilizer for growing vegetables and other plants. If there is an agricultural extension worker in the community, discuss with him how to make compost and how he can help you in persuading households to make it.

Unit 7
Disposal of excreta: latrines

People who have diarrhoea, cholera, or worms pass these diseases on through their faeces. Like waste, faeces attract flies and animals. Flies that land on faeces that contain germs can carry these germs to food, and people who eat such food may fall ill. Therefore, people should not be careless about where they defecate.

If people defecate near a river or spring there is a danger that the water can become dirty, and that people drinking this water may then fall ill.

To prevent the diseases that are spread through faeces, people should not defecate in places where other people, flies, animals and birds can touch the faeces, or where water can be contaminated.

Every household should have a latrine of its own.

If human excreta is left in a pit for 2–3 months it turns into fertilizer. This can be used in the fields to grow plants. If you want to know more about this, ask your supervisor.

Learning objectives

After studying this unit you should be able to:

1 Find out where the village people go to defecate.

2 Discuss with the people why it is dangerous to defecate just anywhere, why a household should build a latrine, and how to do so.

3 Help households to build their own latrines and make sure they use and maintain them properly.

4 Show the people how a latrine should be properly used and maintained.

The problem

Some people in your community defecate carelessly in the open.
Others do not keep their latrines clean. Many children and other
people are suffering from diseases that are carried by faeces. The
people do not know that the way they defecate causes diseases to
spread. What do you do?

First find out where the villagers go to defecate, then discuss why
it is dangerous to defecate just anywhere. The following actions
can be taken depending upon the situation in your community.

When people have no latrines

If people defecate around their houses

There is a danger of disease from faeces, particularly when people
defecate less than 20 metres away from the house or on the paths
that lead to the house.

- Advise the head of the household to tell the family to defecate in
  a latrine or, if they have no latrine, to defecate in the fields away
  from the house.

- Ask for the help of the village chief. He may speak to the people
  about the problem. If he wants the people to build latrines, ask
  your supervisor for help. Afterwards make sure that the latrines
  are being used properly.

If people defecate in the river

The river water becomes dirty and dangerous when people
defecate in it. Tell the people *not to defecate*:

- in the river

- within 20 metres of the river

- on the path leading to the river.

If people continue to do so in spite of your telling them not to, ask
the village chief to help in persuading the people to build latrines
and not to defecate in or around the river.

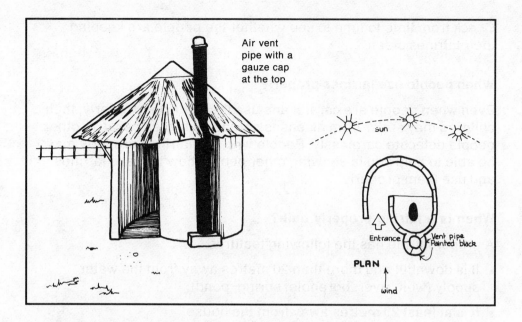

If people defecate in the fields or the forest

There is not much danger of disease if people defecate in the fields or the forest, provided that:

- people defecate at least 20 metres away from any house, spring, well, river, etc.
- people defecate far away from any path or track.

In the open, it is better to defecate in sunny places rather than in the shade. The sun can kill the germs in the faeces. People should not defecate in agricultural fields.

Remember, it is always best to use a latrine, if possible.

When people have latrines but do not use them properly

Advise the head of the household to:

- make sure that no faeces are left on the slab (cover) of the latrines
- have the latrine scrubbed and cleaned regularly with water.

Check from time to time to see whether the people are keeping their latrines clean.

When people use latrines properly

Even when people are careful and use their latrines properly, their children may suffer from diseases spread by faeces because other people defecate carelessly. People who use latrines properly may be able to help you in showing other people how to make latrines and use them properly.

When is a latrine properly built?

A proper latrine has the following features:

- It is downhill and more than 20 metres away from the water supply (well, river, borehole, spring, pond).

- It is at least 20 metres away from the house.

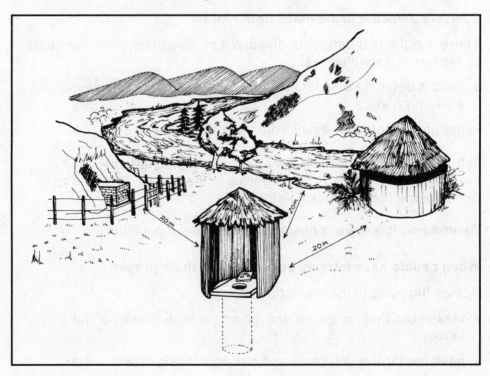

- It has a pit at least 1 metre deep.

- It has a slab (cover) over the pit made of concrete (best) or wood; the slab has a hole through which faeces and urine can drop. The hole should be small enough so that children too can use the latrine; but it should be large enough for faeces and urine to fall through it. The hole should have a cover.

- It has walls and a roof made of materials that are easy to get and cheap to buy and repair.

- It is kept clean. (A separate broom and water bucket should be kept for cleaning the latrine. Water for washing or leaves or paper for cleaning oneself should also be kept in the latrine.)

Other types of latrines can also be built, depending on local conditions. You should discuss this with your supervisor.

When is a latrine properly used?

A latrine is properly used when:

- everyone in the household uses it

- it is kept clean and the floor and the slab are washed often

- the pit is kept covered when the latrine is not being used

- materials for personal cleaning are always available (water, leaves, paper)

- the pit is emptied or a new one is dug when the pit is full.

When a new pit is dug, the latrine is moved to the new site. The earth from the new pit is used to cover the old one, but the same slab is used to keep the new pit covered.

Always remember!

1 *To avoid diseases carried by faeces, people should defecate in a latrine.*

2 *When there are no latrines, people may defecate in a hole far away from the house and from the water supply (village well, river, spring or pond). Cover the hole with earth after defecating.*

3 *Always wash hands with soap and water after defecating.*

Unit 8

Keeping schoolchildren healthy

Children are usually the healthiest group in the community. They are generally interested in new ideas and eager to learn.

It is important to teach children about health care. This is best done by teaching them about everyday life. When schoolchildren learn about health at school they go home and tell their parents what they have learnt. In this way the parents also learn new things about health care.

Children should be encouraged to take part in community health activities. This will increase their interest in health and help them to learn fast.

Learning objectives

After studying this unit, you should be able to:

1 Discuss community health with the village schoolteacher and talk about what each of you can do about health.

2 Exchange information and ideas regularly with the schoolteacher about health and health problems.

3 Report to the community committee about the health of schoolchildren and how to improve it.

Discussion with the schoolteacher

The schoolteacher is a trained person who knows the importance of health and cleanliness. Teachers know that healthy children learn better than sick children. You should offer to help the teacher in keeping the children healthy and in teaching them about health and how to deal with health problems. Often, the teacher will be an influential person in the community and can support you in your health work.

Finding out about the health of schoolchildren

(1) Information about the teacher:

- How long has the teacher been in the community? Is he or she a member of the community committee?

- What can you discuss with the teacher about community life and activities?

- Was health education a part of the teacher's training?

- What does the teacher know about the main health problems in the community, and about what the community is doing to improve health and living standards?

(2) Information about the school:

- Is there a school committee? What does it do? Does it discuss and take action on health activities and health and sanitary facilities in the school?

- Does the school have water for drinking and for washing hands? If not, has anyone talked about providing water at the school?

- Are there latrines at the school? If yes, what is done to keep them clean and safe for everyone? If no, what do children do when they need to use a latrine? Has the community or the school committee discussed this problem?

(3) Information about schoolchildren:

- How many are there? How old are the youngest and oldest children?

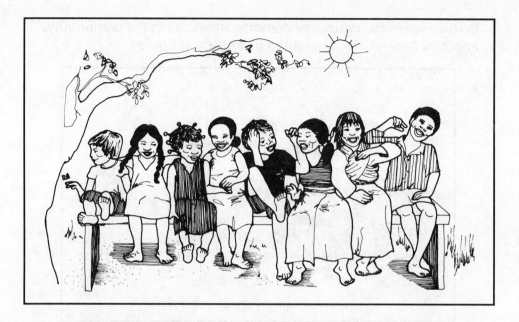

- Has the teacher been able to detect any health problems in the children? What problems have been found?

- What does the teacher do about children with health problems?

- What does the teacher do about children who cannot see well, hear well, or learn well?

Learning about health at school

Find out:

- What do the children learn at school about health?

- Do they learn ways of protecting themselves against illnesses? For example, do they know: why and how latrines should be built and used? Why it is important to be immunized? Why it is important to be clean? Do they learn how to clean their teeth after meals?

- Do they learn practical ways of being healthy, such as how to grow food that is good for health and how to prepare it? Do they learn how to prevent accidents and treat common injuries?

■ Do they learn the causes of common illnesses in the community and how they can be prevented or treated at home?

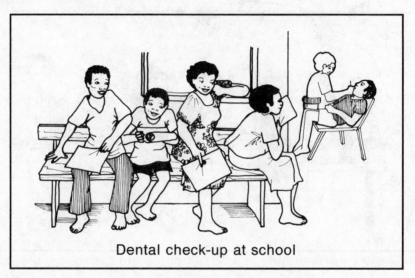

Dental check-up at school

The teacher should know about you and your work

It will be useful if you discuss the above questions with the teacher. This will show that you are concerned about the children's health. The teacher will then understand that you are there to help the people to improve their own health.

With your help and with the help of the teacher, the children will be able to learn how to care for themselves.

When you and the teacher work together, you will be better able to convince the community about what can be done at school to make the community more healthy, and how the school and you can work together to improve the health of the children and their families.

What can be done to improve the health of schoolchildren?

Try to give advice if the teacher asks you about the children's health. Show the teacher this book or any other health book you have. Ask your supervisor about problems you cannot solve yourself.

List the problems at the school, for example:

- There may be no water for drinking or for washing hands.
- The school may need a first-aid box and supplies.
- The school may need money to make a vegetable garden or to raise poultry.
- The children may need latrines, or the existing latrines may need to be kept cleaner.

Decide together with the teacher which problem should be dealt with first.

Tell the teacher about the health problems in the community as they happen. For example, if a lot of people get diarrhoea, the children should be taught how to make a solution from salt, sugar, and water (oral rehydration solution; see Unit 26). They should know why this solution is useful, and how to give it to children with diarrhoea. If there is malaria in the district, the children can be trained to destroy breeding-places of mosquitos (see Unit 9), to take antimalarial tablets at school, and to make mosquito nets.

Ask the teacher to report to the school committee or the community committee on what you have discussed and agreed upon, so that the committee can take action.

Arrange to meet the teacher regularly to discuss health problems of schoolchildren.

Always remember!

Before starting any health or community development work involving schoolchildren, discuss the subject with the schoolteacher and get his or her agreement (see Unit 1).

Unit 9
Vectors of disease

A vector is an animal that passes a disease from one animal or person to another animal or person.

Many serious illnesses are passed on to humans by vectors such as:

- *insects (e.g., mosquitos, flies)*
- *animals that live in water (e.g., snails)*
- *land animals (e.g., rats and dogs).*

You should learn from your supervisor which vectors are common in your area, and inform him about the cases of diseases caused by them.

The CHW should collect information on diseases spread by vectors and pass it on to community leaders so that they can decide what to do to prevent as many of these diseases as possible.

Learning objectives

After studying this unit, you should be able to:

1 Explain to the people in your area the dangers of vectors of disease (some insects and animals).

2 Identify the places where these vectors live and breed, and explain how to fight against them.

3 Discuss with families and with various groups in the community what they might do to reduce contact between people and vectors.

4 Tell them what the health services are doing to fight various vectors of disease in the community.

Fevers and diseases are passed on by vectors in your area

In many parts of the world, and particularly in hot countries, many insects and animals, e.g., mosquitos, flies, snails, rats, dogs, can carry diseases, which they may pass on to people.

Insects

Mosquitos can carry malaria and other diseases such as yellow fever, dengue fever, haemorrhagic fever, and filariasis. Houseflies can carry the germs of diarrhoea. Blackflies carry small worms which form lumps under the skin and cause river blindness.

Water animals

Snails that live in water can carry small worms (blood flukes), which can get into the water and pass through the skin of people who swim or wash or walk there. These worms cause blood in the urine (schistosomiasis).

Land animals

Rats carry diseases. They may bite humans and other animals, and contaminate food. In this way they pass on fevers and other severe diseases. Bites of sick dogs can be very dangerous, as they may pass on rabies. To protect against rat and dog bites, see Unit 34.

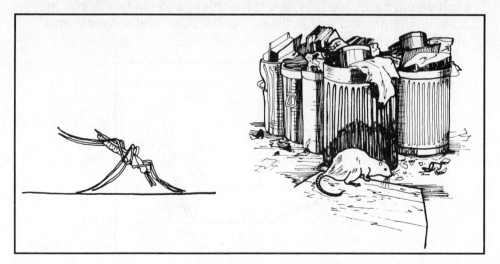

Find out from your supervisor what are the common vectors of fevers and other diseases in your area. Ask which of these fevers and other diseases you can help to prevent.

Fighting against vectors of fevers and other diseases

Destroying or limiting the breeding-places of vectors

Mosquitos breed and multiply in standing water. They can breed even in small amounts of rainwater that collect in old tin cans, old tyres, small holes in the ground or in trees, etc. Always remember that, where there are mosquitos, any water collected in open holes, vessels, old tyres, cans, etc., is a danger to health.

Flies breed on all kinds of waste and rubbish and in animal and human excreta (see Units 6 and 7). Blackflies, the vectors of river blindness, breed in running water (streams and rivers).

If you know where vectors breed, you can destroy their breeding-places and thereby destroy the vectors. You should work together with the people and continuously destroy the breeding-places of the vectors in your community and prevent new ones from being made. Give the people the following advice:

- Remind everybody in the community (including children and old people) that mosquitos breed in rainwater that collects in things such as old cans, old jars, broken bottles, and old tyres, and in holes in the ground and in trees, ponds, open wells, lakes, and marshes (swamps).

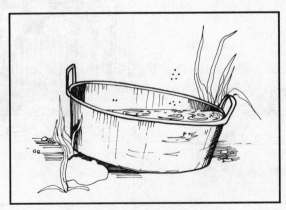

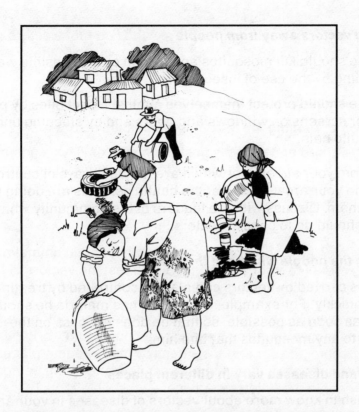

Ask the people to look for such places and get rid of them. For example, they can burn coconut shells. If they keep water in jars, they should empty the jars every 2–3 days so that they do not become breeding-places. If there are many old cans and bottles in the rubbish, ask the people to bury such rubbish. In the case of old tyres, people can make holes in them so that water does not collect in them.

- People should make sure that their latrines are kept clean and the pits are kept covered when not in use (see Unit 7).

- Wells and springs should be kept covered (see Unit 4).

- Advise the people to fill in or treat ponds, pools or ditches where mosquitos and snails can breed. Ask your supervisor about ways of treating ponds and ditches.

Keeping vectors away from people

- People should kill mosquitos and flies in every possible way, including by the use of insecticides.

- People should protect themselves against insect bites by putting nets or screens on windows and doors and by sleeping under mosquito nets.

Learn from your supervisor which are the best ways of controlling vectors in your area, and what the health services are doing to control them. Discuss with the leaders of the community what the people should do to control vectors.

Treating the people who have the diseases

Diseases carried by vectors can also be controlled by treating sick people quickly. For example, if a person has malaria he should be treated as soon as possible, so that he does not pass on the disease to any mosquitos that bite him.

Vectors and diseases vary in different places

If you wish to know more about vectors of diseases in your area you should ask your supervisor; he or she may give you other books to read.

Schistosomiasis (blood in urine). Snails are the vectors of this disease. People get this disease when they wash or swim in water that has snails. Little worms come out of the snails and enter the body through the skin. Inside the body they breed and produce schistosomiasis, in which there is blood in the urine. A person who has this disease has eggs of the worms in his urine and faeces. When such a person urinates or defecates in a pond or lake where there are snails, the eggs get into the snails and become worms. These worms can then cause the disease in other people who wash or swim in that water. You should ask people not to urinate or defecate in ponds and lakes.

Other vectors living in the water may carry guinea-worm disease (dracunculosis). In countries where guinea worms are common the people should drink water only from safe places, where there are no vectors. If the water is not safe, they should always filter it through a cloth or through a filter of fine sand to remove the larvae of guinea worms (see Annex 2, section 7).

Sleeping sickness. If you live in a country where sleeping sickness occurs, you should know that the *tsetse fly* carries and passes on this disease to people. You will have to learn about the tsetse fly, and the parts of the body on which it bites. To catch and kill this fly you should know how to make and set up simple fly traps in your area (see picture below).

How to make a tsetse-fly trap

1 The trap is made up of two conical parts fixed to a rigid frame. The top part is made of thin white material, and the bottom part

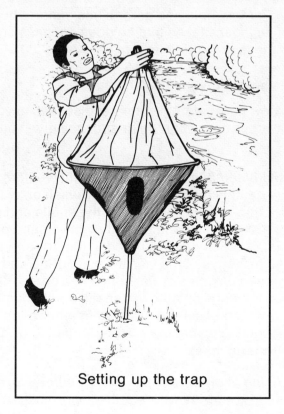

Setting up the trap

75

is made of material which is blue on the outside and black inside.

2 The white part is closed at the top and is soaked with insecticide.

3 There are four holes in the bottom part.

4 Tsetse flies are attracted by the colours of the trap and enter it through the holes.

5 Once inside the trap, they are attracted by the daylight coming through the white part and they fly upwards where they are killed by the insecticide.

Chapter 3
Keeping the family healthy

Unit 10
Personal and family hygiene

As a community health worker you should set an example of healthy living and good health in the community. The community will then imitate your habits.

People will learn healthy habits by watching how you live and look after your family and house.

Cleanliness is the most basic health habit.

Learning objectives

After studying this unit you should be able to:

1 Set an example of good personal hygiene and healthy living in your community.

2 Discuss with families how healthy habits prevent diseases.

3 Discuss with people why cigarette smoking and tobacco chewing are bad for health.

4 Discuss with people why clean water is essential for health.

5 Discuss with people why spitting is a dirty habit.

6 Discuss with people why they should always wear shoes.

You and your family should have healthy habits:

(1) Look clean.

(2) Wash your hands before and after meals, and keep your fingernails short and clean.

(3) Do not smoke cigarettes or chew tobacco.

(4) Boil the water to prepare feeds for small children.

(5) Use a safe bathing place.

(6) Clean your teeth after meals.

(7) Have one or more latrines, which all members of the family use.

(8) Never urinate or defecate anywhere on the ground or in water.

(9) Do not spit on the ground.

(10) Wear shoes or sandals that are made or obtained locally (see Unit 38).

(11) Never drink too much alcohol. It is best not to drink alcohol at all.

Ask yourself questions about healthy habits

■ How do my health habits affect my health and that of my family?

■ If everyone had my habits, would the health of the community improve?

It is important for you to have healthy habits. You will learn these during training. You must set an example of healthy living in your community. If you do not have healthy habits yourself, you will not be able to advise others to change their unhealthy ways of living.

Ask yourself: how do I look?

Your appearance will show what you think of yourself. If you do not look clean and healthy, you will find it hard to be an effective community health worker.

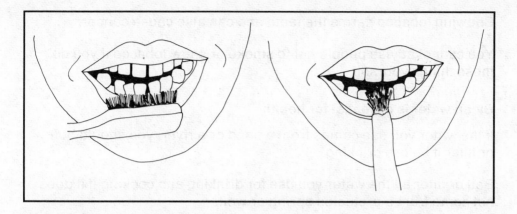

Do you brush or clean your teeth after every meal? Advise others to do this as well. Discuss with people why it is a good habit to clean the teeth after meals.

Washing hands is important

You and your family may catch diseases or pass diseases on to other people if you do not all keep your hands clean.

Food prepared with dirty hands can carry diseases.

Even if water is scarce, try to wash hands with soap and water at least before you prepare and eat food, and after defecating.

Discuss with people how they can prevent diseases by keeping their hands clean.

Smoking cigarettes and chewing tobacco harms health

Do not smoke. Cigarette smoke harms your lungs and your family's lungs.

It may cause coughing and yellow sputum. Smoking cigarettes can also cause serious diseases such as cancer.

Chewing tobacco harms the teeth and can also cause cancer.

You cannot advise people not to smoke or chew tobacco if you do these things yourself.

Clean water is essential for health

If the water you use comes from a pond or a river, you should boil or filter it before drinking.

Boil or filter all the water you use for drinking and cooking if it does not come from a protected spring or well.

Learn to filter the water and to keep the filter clean (see section 7 in Annex 2). Also, you can add bleaching powder to the water after you filter it.

Bathing

You and your family should bathe in a safe place where the water flows rapidly and no plants are growing. It is a good idea to have a bathroom in the house if people can afford it. If you use soap, you will need less water and your skin will be cleaner.

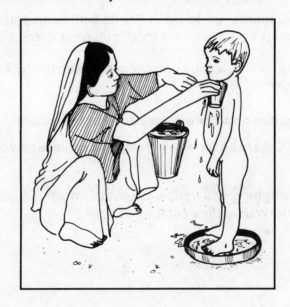

80

Have a latrine at or near your house and use it properly (see Unit 7).

Never urinate or defecate in water, or on damp ground.

If your children learn the habit of always using a latrine when they are young, they and their children will not have the problems of worms.

Never spit carelessly

Spitting is a bad habit. Spit contains germs that can cause disease. Advise people not to spit on the ground.

When you have to spit, you should spit into a special cloth or a container. Keep the container clean by washing it regularly.

Use simple, locally made shoes or sandals

Some worms (hookworms) enter the body through the feet (see Unit 38). This can be prevented by wearing shoes. If you wear simple, locally made shoes, others can more easily imitate what you do than if you wear expensive shoes.

Encourage people to wear shoes.

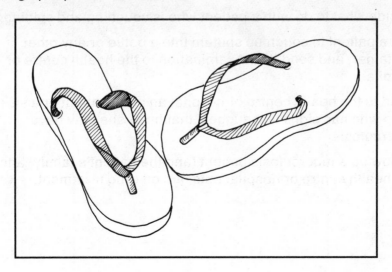

Unit 11
Tuberculosis

Tuberculosis (TB) is a chronic disease. This means it can go on for several months or even a few years if it is not treated at all or if it is not treated properly.

Tuberculosis usually affects the lungs and causes the patient to cough and spit. In severe cases it causes the patient to cough up blood. In children and young people it can affect the bones, brain, and other organs.

Everybody should know that tuberculosis is dangerous, and may cause death. It can spread from one person to others. The people need to know that patients with tuberculosis can be cured with drugs, and that the disease can be prevented.

Learning objectives

After studying this unit, you should be able to:

1 Explain to the people how tuberculosis is spread and how to prevent it.

2 Decide what to do with a patient who is coughing and spitting.

3 Ask a patient to cough up sputum into a bottle or any other container, and send it for examination to the health centre or hospital.

4 Send to the health centre or hospital an adult patient or a sick child who has signs that suggest that he or she may have tuberculosis.

5 Follow up a tuberculosis patient (and the patient's family) after the health centre or hospital puts him on drug treatment.

How tuberculosis spreads and how it can be prevented

How people catch tuberculosis

When people live or work with other people who have tuberculosis of the lungs and who are coughing and spitting there is a danger of catching tuberculosis. A patient who coughs can spread the germs of tuberculosis into the air. Other people who breathe the same air can breathe in the germs, and in this way catch the disease. This disease is especially dangerous to young children who have not been immunized with BCG vaccine, and to other non-immunized people who are weak and badly fed.

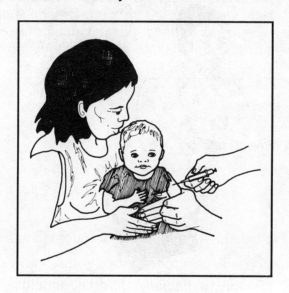

How to prevent tuberculosis in your community

Explain to the people that:

- All newborn babies and young children should be immunized against tuberculosis with the BCG vaccine. This may cause a slight wound which will heal without any treatment. The vaccine gives good protection.

- Anyone who has a cough for more than three weeks and who coughs up and spits blood, and has pain in the chest or difficulty in breathing should come to see you. You should send such a

83

patient to the health centre or hospital. After that person returns from hospital, visit him regularly to make sure that he is taking the medicine as told by the doctor.

■ People who have TB should cover their mouth with a handkerchief when they cough and should not spit on the ground. They should spit into an old cloth or paper or leaf or anything else that can be burned after use.

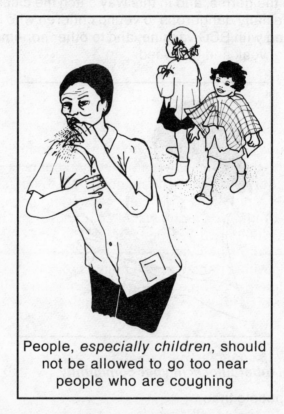

People, *especially children*, should
not be allowed to go too near
people who are coughing

What to do with a patient who is coughing and spitting

If the patient has been coughing and spitting for less than three weeks

(1) If there is fever (see Unit 24),

■ advise the patient to rest for a few days

- give aspirin for 3–5 days (see Annex 1, Medicines).

(2) If there is no fever,

- advise the patient to rest for a few days and to keep warm.

After 3–5 days, the patient should have improved and you do not need to do anything else. If there is no improvement, send him to the health centre or hospital.

If the patient has been coughing and spitting for more than three weeks

This could be a serious illness. Always send this patient to the health centre or hospital, and ask him to come back to see you afterwards.

If the patient does not or cannot go to the health centre or hospital, ask him to cough up some sputum into a clean bottle or jar, write his name and address on the bottle, and send it to the health centre or hospital for examination. The health centre should send you the results of the examination along with a supply of drugs to treat the patient and the family, and instructions on how to take the drugs.

People who live with a patient who coughs and spits may catch the illness. They should also be examined at the health centre and told to come to see you if they have fever or if they start coughing and spitting.

Other people with coughing illness who must go to the health centre or hospital at once

Send to the health centre or hospital:

(1) any person who:

- has blood in his sputum
- has a bad smell in his sputum
- has lost weight
- feels hot and sweats a lot at night

(2) any person who has a coughing disease, with or without any of the above signs, and who is working or has worked in a dusty job (for example, in a mine, gravel works, construction site, quarry)

(3) any child or young person who has been unwell for a few weeks and has some or all of the following signs:

- is always tired

- does not want to play or work

- does not want to eat

- is becoming thin

- is sometimes feverish

- sometimes has a bad cough.

Find out from the health centre if these people have tuberculosis. Visit them regularly to make sure that they are taking their medicines properly.

In the case of a young person or a child, apart from visiting him or her regularly, you will have to ask for your supervisor's help in finding out from whom the child got the disease. Also, see which other children are in danger of catching the disease from the same person. Ask your supervisor what else you can do.

Advise the family of the child on how to look after him. Also, tell the schoolteacher about the disease. The child may have given the disease to other children at school.

Follow up a TB patient and the patient's family

When a TB patient comes back home from the health centre or hospital, he should bring with him enough medicines to last several months and instructions on how to take them. Ask him to show you these.

Explain to the patient that if he wants to get well he must take the medicines regularly.

Visit the patient every 2 or 3 weeks to make sure that he is taking the medicines as prescribed. Ask the family to help him to remember to do so and to check that he does take them. Also remind the patient when he will have to go back to the health centre or hospital for check ups (usually every 3 months).

Make sure that any children and young persons living or working with a TB patient are immunized against TB, and are examined at the health centre or hospital if they start coughing and spitting.

Unit 12
Chronic illness

A chronic illness is one that lasts a long time. An illness that is not coming to an end after about three months may be said to be chronic.

It causes long suffering for the person who is ill and usually causes problems for the family members who may have to support and care for the patient.

It usually prevents the person from living a normal life.

Chronic illness can disable a person for the rest of his life (see also Unit 14). It may even lead to death.

Learning objectives

After studying this unit you should be able to:

1 Identify people in the community who have chronic illnesses and need care.

2 Refer chronically ill patients to a health centre for diagnosis and treatment.

3 Advise and help the family on how to look after a chronically ill person who:

- is able to move around by himself
- is unable to move around without support
- is lying in bed all the time.

4 Encourage and advise a chronically ill patient to continue as much as he can with the usual activities of daily living.

88

Signs of chronic illness

A person suffering from a long illness of the body or mind may always feel weak and tired, and may spend most of the time in bed.

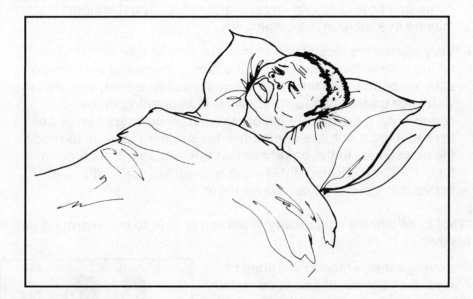

Some of the other signs of common chronic illnesses are:

- chronic cough and fever
- pain in different parts of the body
- chronic diarrhoea
- difficulty in passing urine
- abnormal colour of the skin, or other symptoms.

A chronically ill person may not be able to walk easily because his legs may be weak, deformed, painful, or swollen.

How you can help a person with chronic illness

- Arrange with the family to take the patient to a health centre for diagnosis and any treatment that may be needed.

■ Visit the patient regularly and make sure that the patient and the family can do what the doctor or nurse has advised, and that the patient takes the prescribed medicine regularly.

■ Advise and guide the family on how to look after the patient at home and how to obtain any social or educational support that may be available in the community.

■ Very often, chronically ill persons are very lonely. Apart from taking care of the basic needs, the family members may not be able to spend much time with them. If you have time, you should visit such people and tell them what is happening in the community. If the patient is able to read, encourage him or her to read a lot. If not, ask someone who is willing to help, to read the newspaper to the patient or just talk with him from time to time. Keeping chronically ill people cheerful, optimistic, and active is the best you can do for them.

What to do when a chronically ill person is able to move around on his own

Encourage the person to continue to carry out all the usual activities of daily living he or she is able to do, for example:

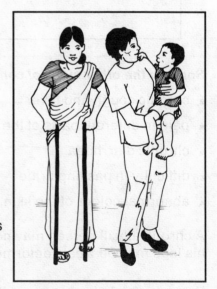

■ taking part in normal family life and helping with household tasks

■ continuing with normal work (if it is not too tiring)

■ taking part in social activities

■ in the case of a child, going to school; you should discuss the needs and limitations of such a child with the schoolteachers.

What to do when a chronically ill person is not able to move around

Discuss with the family what they can do to encourage and help the patient to look after his own needs, such as eating and drinking, washing and keeping clean, dressing and undressing, and other activities.

When the person is very weak and lying in bed all the time

When a person is so weak and ill that he cannot even change his position in bed by himself, he can easily get bedsores and infections of the lungs. Also, the arms and legs may become bent and useless.

Discuss with the family how they can:

- keep the patient and his bed and bedclothes clean

- change the position of the patient in the bed every few hours so that he never lies for long in the same position

- protect with soft padding or pillows the parts of the body that easily get bedsores (see drawing)

- take the person out of the bed for some time once or twice every day (make him sit, stand, or take a few steps, depending on his condition)

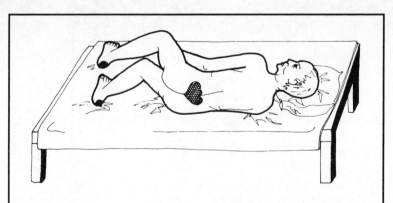

Patients who lie in bed all the time and who are weak and sick can easily get bed sores on parts of the body where the bones are covered only by skin.

91

- move the arms and legs as fully as possible several times a day
- encourage the patient to move his body, arms and legs as much as possible
- make sure that the patient takes enough fluid and food.

Unit 13
Health care of old people

> *Old people have a right to health care and to enjoy old age.*
>
> *You can make use of the experience, wisdom, and remaining activity of old people to improve the health of the community.*

Learning objectives

After studying this unit you should be able to:

1 Describe to the people the three important factors that can help make life longer.

2 Recognize and treat the common health problems of old people.

3 Advise old people to make use of the three levels of care.

4 Involve old people in health activities.

Three important factors that contribute to a long and healthy life

Remind old people and their families that the following three factors can contribute to a healthy and long life:

(1) *Activity*. Elderly people who remain active members of the family and community will feel useful and interested in life. This will help to keep them healthy. They may take more time than others to do what they have to do, but the family should understand this and be patient with them.

(2) *A good diet*. Eating well and regularly is essential for good health.

(3) *Avoiding all excesses*. Too much rest, too much exercise, too much alcohol and too much food are some of the excesses to be avoided.

Common health problems of old people

In addition to providing primary care to sick elderly people, the CHW should also try to detect and follow up special problems of old age. These are mostly related to the eyes, ears, joints, passing urine, and loss of memory.

The eyes

Most elderly people need glasses to read or see things in detail. Some will need an eye operation if they are gradually losing their sight and if they complain of cloudy vision (as if they are looking through a fog). This disease is called cataract.

The ears

Some old people cannot hear well. They may be deaf because the ears are blocked by wax, or because of a disease inside the ears. You should send such persons to the health centre for examination and, if necessary, to have wax taken out. Some deaf elderly persons can be helped with a hearing-aid or with an ear-trumpet.

Painful joints

This is a common problem in old people. See Unit 29 for instructions on how to help old people with painful joints.

Problems related to passing urine

When an old man cannot urinate easily or if the urine drips or dribbles, this probably means that his prostate gland has enlarged. Refer him to the health centre or hospital as he may need an operation to remove it.

Old women may not be able to hold their urine, and the urine may dribble all the time and wet their clothes. Their bodies will smell of stale urine. If they cannot care for themselves, they will need continuous personal care to keep clean. Sometimes an operation in hospital can cure or improve their condition. Refer such patients to the health centre or hospital.

Loss of memory and strange behaviour

Old people may gradually lose their memory, become confused, and say and do strange things. There is no medicine that can cure this condition, but a balanced diet together with family care, love, kindness, and patience will help to prevent the old person's state of mind from getting worse too quickly.

Sometimes the confusion appears very quickly, and the skin may become dry and cracked at the same time. This is caused by poor nutrition, especially if the diet is mostly rice or corn. Also, sometimes an old person may become confused suddenly because of an infection with fever.

The three levels of health care

(1) *Self care*. Everybody should look after his or her own health. Old people should be particularly encouraged to do so because this is the best way of remaining active. The less the old people depend on other people, the better it will be for them and for their families.

(2) *Family care*. Many old people are unable to do everything for themselves. Families of old people should help them with things that they cannot do.

(3) *Community care*. Sometimes all members of the family may have to go out to work, leaving an old person at home. If this

elderly person cannot manage on his own, other members of the community can help by preparing meals or doing other things for him. Old people who live alone may also need this type of help. The CHW is responsible for treating common health problems of the aged and helping families to look after themselves better.

Involving old people in health activities

Try to benefit from the experience of old people. They know a lot about the community. Some may know local traditional ways of treating some injuries or symptoms. They may be able to give you good advice.

Try to involve them in some of your activities, for example by asking them to look after your health post, to visit other old people, to take part in the community committee, or in any other way that makes them feel useful.

Disabled people

Disabled people are persons who:

- *are deaf or cannot hear well*
- *are blind or cannot see well*
- *are paralysed or cannot move easily*
- *cannot speak or speak poorly*
- *cannot learn easily*
- *cannot feel heat or cold or pain or touch in their hands or feet.*

Disabled people often depend on their families or other people for feeding, dressing, using a latrine, and getting from one place to another. Such people can be trained to reduce or overcome their disabilities and to take an active part in the community.

Learning objectives

After studying this unit you should be able to:

1 Identify disabled persons in your community, and, if possible, keep a list of them.

2 Discuss with them, their families, and your supervisor how their disability may be reduced by training at home.

3 Send to the health centre or hospital only those disabled persons who can benefit from treatment to reduce their disability.

Identifying and helping disabled people

Some disabled people live fairly normal lives in their families and can make a living. They will not need any special treatment. Others may need training to overcome or reduce their disability.

In some cases the disability can be cured or very much improved. For example:

- A person who has poor sight may be able to see well with proper glasses or may be cured by a small operation.

- A person who is deaf or cannot hear well may be cured by an operation or may be able to hear with an ear-trumpet or a hearing-aid, or may learn to lip-read.

- A person who cannot move at all or cannot move easily can sometimes be trained to walk with crutches or to move around in a wheelchair.

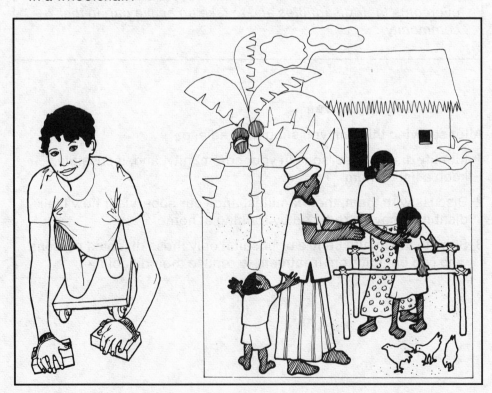

- A person who cannot eat or drink without help may be able to use special spoons, cups, or plates.

- A person who cannot look after himself or herself may be trained by another family member to eat, drink, wash, use the latrine, and do other tasks of daily living.

- A person who cannot speak may be trained with the help of other family members to communicate by means of sign language.

If your community is in a town or city, you should find out where disabled people can be trained and arrange for disabled persons in your area to follow such a training, if possible.

A disabled mother can be trained to wash her hands and her breasts and to feed her baby and care for it. She can be trained to cook food for her children and wash them. Also, in some places, a family member can be trained to help a disabled person to care for himself or to do certain kinds of work.

A family member can be trained to help a child who cannot see well, or hear well, or speak well, or use a spoon or a cup or a pencil, or learn easily, or keep himself clean.

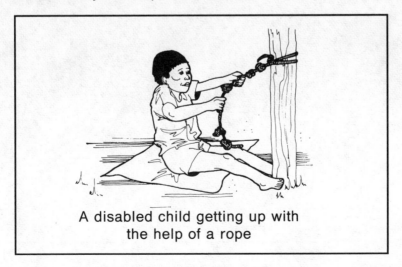

A disabled child getting up with
the help of a rope

If you cannot send disabled people for training in your area, try to contact an institution or a centre that trains disabled people in another area, and ask for its advice.

Whenever possible, disabled persons should be examined in a health centre or hospital to see whether they can have treatment or special care, or whether they can be trained or helped to do things so that they can lead a more normal life.

Ask your supervisor's advice on how to train disabled persons in your community. Discuss with the community committee or with a women's group how to help disabled people to live a normal life (see also Units 13, 29, and 37).

Chapter 4

Health care of women

Unit 15
Pregnancy

Some community health workers are trained to provide care
for pregnant women or assist at childbirth and some are not.
If you are trained to do so, you should always keep in mind
that some women may prefer to be cared for by the
traditional birth attendant (TBA) or the nurse/midwife. In
such cases you should attend a delivery only if the woman
wants you to do so.

When you begin work in a community you should visit the
TBA and the nurse/midwife. Tell them about the work you
are going to do in the community. Offer to share with them
your information and knowledge so that by working together
you can help the community to improve its hygiene and
health, particularly the health of mothers and children.

Learning objectives

After studying this unit you should be able to:

1 Explain to a woman how she becomes pregnant and how the
baby grows inside her body.

2 Explain to mothers the risk factors that may make pregnancy
dangerous for the mother and the baby.

3 Find out if a woman is pregnant or not. Identify pregnant women
who need to visit the health centre soon and explain to them and
their families why they need to do so.

4 Recognize serious problems in pregnancy and begin treatment;
discuss with a family why the woman must go for treatment to a
hospital or health centre, and help the family to arrange for her
to go.

5 Discuss with a family what can be done to protect and improve the health of the pregnant woman and her unborn baby.

6 Discuss with the community committee and other groups and leaders the needs and problems of pregnant women and help them to decide on community action to protect and improve the health of pregnant women.

7 Collect information about pregnant women in the community, and use this information in your work.

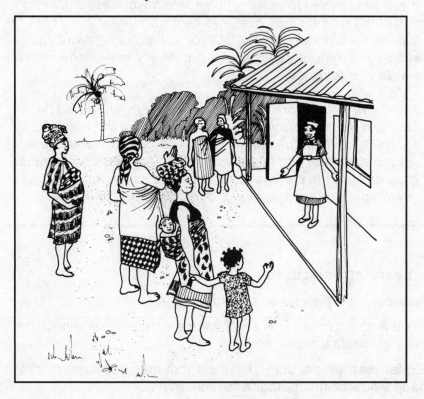

Facts about pregnancy

Before a pregnancy can begin, the woman must be producing **eggs**[1] in her body and the man producing **sperm** in his.

When a young woman begins to lose blood regularly every month (at about 14 years of age), this means her body is making eggs. This blood loss is often called a **period**.

When a man's sperm enters a woman's body it may join with one of the woman's eggs; she then becomes pregnant. Then her periods will stop and a baby will begin to grow in her womb (**uterus**).

A woman, between 14 and 45 years of age, who has not had a period for 6–8 weeks or more is probably pregnant.

After a woman has been pregnant for three months, the **placenta** (or afterbirth) is formed in her womb. The placenta is connected to the baby's body at the navel by a cord (**umbilical cord**). Some of the food that the mother eats goes to the placenta to nourish the baby. If the mother does not eat enough food, the baby cannot get enough from the placenta and will not grow to a normal size and weight.

A person who works hard needs a lot of food. A pregnant woman who works too hard uses all her food to do her work. This leaves too little to go to the placenta for the baby. To make sure that a baby will grow well and be strong, all pregnant women should rest more and do less work than usual.

Nine months after the last normal period, the baby is ready to live outside the mother's body. To let the baby out the womb begins to open. This is called **labour**.

Risk factors in pregnancy

A risk factor is something that increases danger to health. There are certain risk factors in pregnancy. You should look for the

---

[1] See glossary on page 415 for words you cannot understand.

following risk factors in the women in your community. Any of them can make a pregnancy more dangerous than usual for the mother and the baby. Advise women about the dangers before they become pregnant.

Risk factor no. 1

The woman is less than 17 years old.

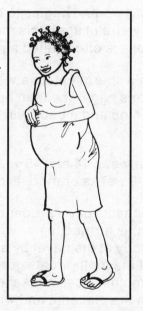

Risk factor no. 2

She already has more than 5 children.

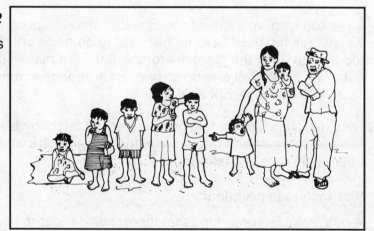

Risk factor no. 3

Her last baby was
born less than two
years ago.

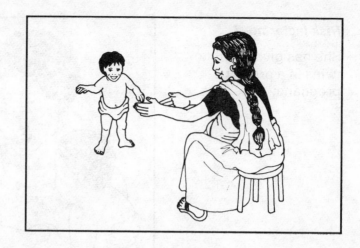

Risk factor no. 4

She had severe bleeding during her last pregnancy.

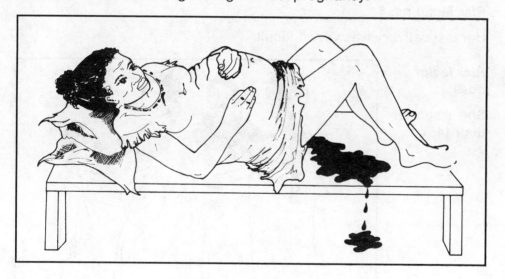

Risk factor no. 5

Her last baby was born dead or died soon after birth.

Risk factor no. 6

Her last baby was very small and weighed less than 2.5 kg at birth.

Risk factor no. 7

She has given birth to twins in a previous pregnancy.

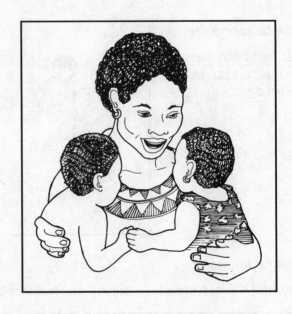

Risk factor no. 8

Her last delivery was very difficult.

Risk factor no. 9

She is shorter than 145 cm.

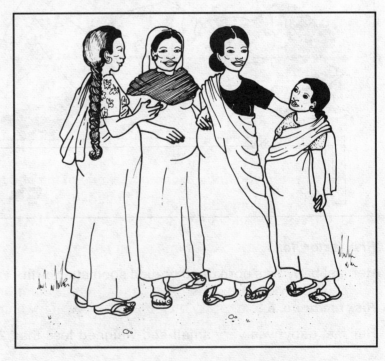

Risk factor no. 10

She weighs less than 45 kg or more than 80 kg.

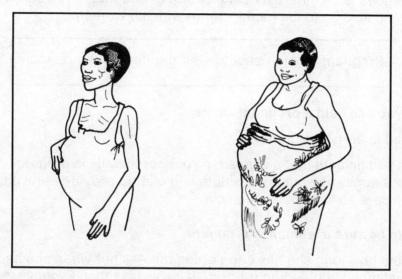

Risk factor no. 11

She is very pale and looks tired.

Risk factor no. 12

She has tuberculosis (TB), malaria, **diabetes**, heart disease, or kidney disease, or she has had an abdominal (belly) operation.

What to do when you find a woman with one of the above factors

When you find a woman between 14 and 45 years old with any of the above risk factors you must:

- Explain to her and to her family about the risks that could be involved in a pregnancy.

- Discuss ways of preventing pregnancy until a safer time, if the risk factor is a temporary one. For example, if a woman is weak and pale, she should not become pregnant until she is strong and healthy.

■ If the woman is pregnant, explain to her and her family that she needs to be seen by the midwife, or arrange with the family that she goes to the nearest health centre or hospital. If you can, you should also go to the health centre with the woman.

> Pregnant women should visit the health centre soon.

How you can help a pregnant woman

Women in early pregnancy

When you find out that a woman in your community is pregnant, visit the family as soon as possible and offer to provide her with health care during the pregnancy.

How to be sure a woman is pregnant

Find out how long she has been pregnant. Ask her when she had her last monthly bleeding (period). If it was less than 2 months ago, tell her that it is too early to be sure that she is pregnant. See her again after 1 month.

If her last bleeding was more than 3 months ago:

■ Ask her to go to the latrine and pass urine. Once the bladder is empty, the womb will be easier to feel.

■ Ask her to lie down. Press your hand gently on the lower belly. If you feel something hard and round, it means that the woman is pregnant. The hard round thing that you felt is her womb (uterus).

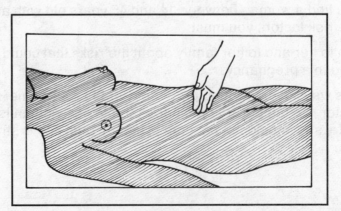

How to tell when the baby will be born

Ask her the date of the first day of her last period. If she does not know use the following picture to tell her when the baby will be born.

If the woman uses a calendar and knows the date of the first day of her last period, you can calculate the date on which the baby will probably be born. This is the expected date of delivery.

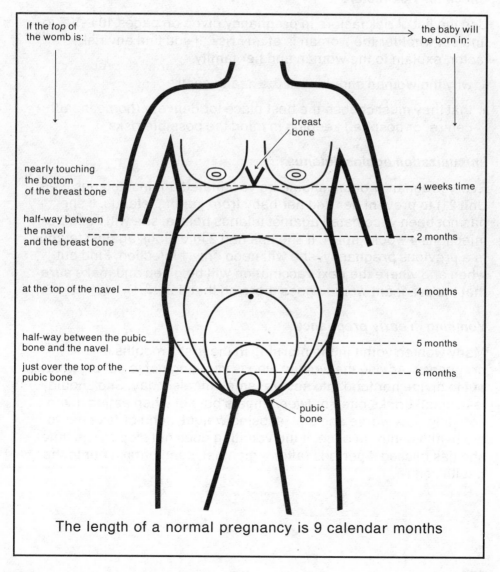

If the *top* of the womb is: ———————————————→ the baby will be born in:

nearly touching the bottom of the breast bone — — — — — — 4 weeks time

breast bone

half-way between the navel and the breast bone — — — — — 2 months

at the top of the navel ————————————— 4 months

half-way between the pubic bone and the navel — — — — — 5 months

just over the top of the pubic bone — — — — — 6 months

pubic bone

The length of a normal pregnancy is 9 calendar months

Add one week to the date of the first day of the last period, and then add nine calendar months to that date.

Example: First day of last period – 5 February
Add one week (7 days) – 12 February
Add nine months   – 12 November is the expected date

Check for risk factors

Use the list of risk factors in pregnancy given on pages 104–107 to find out whether the woman is at any risk. If you find any risk factor, explain to the woman and her family:

- why the woman should visit the health centre
- that they must choose the best place for delivery (home, health centre, or hospital) keeping in mind the possible risks.

Immunization against tetanus

Every pregnant woman should be vaccinated against tetanus (see Unit 21) to prevent her and her baby from getting tetanus. If she has not been vaccinated against tetanus before, she will need 2 injections 4 weeks apart. If she has had 2 injections against tetanus in a previous pregnancy, she will need only 1 injection. Find out when and where the next vaccination will be given and make sure that the pregnant woman goes there on that day.

Vomiting in early pregnancy

Many women vomit in the morning in the first 3 months of pregnancy. Advise the woman who is vomiting not to eat big meals, but to divide her food into several small meals a day. She should take small drinks often *between* meals but not when eating. If the vomiting gets worse and she is losing weight, send or take her to the health centre at once. If the vomiting does not stop by the time she has missed 4 periods (after 4 months), send or take her to the health centre.

Swollen feet

Women's feet may swell, especially in the last three months of pregnancy. To find out whether the feet are swollen, press the skin around each ankle with the thumb (see drawing). If the point at which you pressed becomes a small pit or hollow which does not go away quickly, the feet are swollen.

If the woman has no other problem, advise her:

- to rest with her feet up
- not to add extra salt to her food
- to see you in one week.

If after one week the swelling has not gone, she should go to the health centre.

If a woman with swollen feet also has swelling of the hands and face, headaches, belly pains or pain behind the eyes, she should see the doctor or go to the health centre or hospital at once. This condition can be serious.

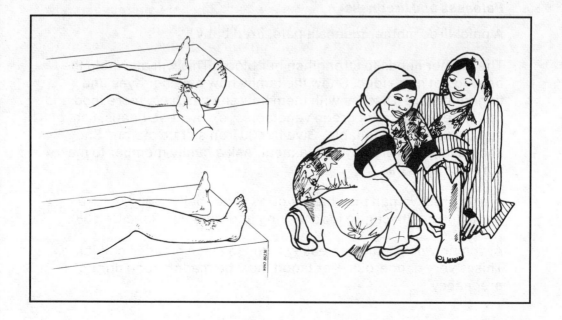

Headache

Many people get headaches when they are hungry or too hot or they have worked too hard. Check that this is not the case with the pregnant woman. Talk to the family to make sure that she is allowed to do less work and to have a little more to eat.

Make sure she has no swelling of her feet or hands (see above). If she has no swelling give her two aspirins and ask the family to let her sleep.

If a woman has headache and swollen feet, this may be dangerous. Give her two aspirins and take her to the health centre.

Fever

Pregnancy does not cause fever. A high fever in pregnancy can be dangerous for the mother and for the baby. Treat the fever according to instructions in Unit 24.

If the fever does not go away in 2 days or gets worse, send or take her to the health centre.

Paleness and tiredness

A pale, tired mother means a pale, tired baby.

The mother needs to strengthen her blood. This will also help the baby to get more food. Show the family how pale her eyes and fingernails are. Discuss with them how she can have more food and rest. She needs more green vegetables, extra meat, beans, fish, or eggs, and milk if available. Give her 30 iron sulfate tablets. She should take 1 every day with a meal. Ask a family member to make sure she does this.

A pale tired woman may have worms in her belly. Send or take her to the health centre for checking and treatment (see Unit 38).

A woman who is pale can easily lose too much blood in childbirth. This is very dangerous. Her blood must be made strong during pregnancy.

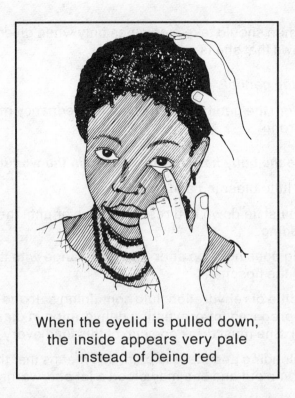

When the eyelid is pulled down,
the inside appears very pale
instead of being red

Recognizing serious problems and starting treatment

General conditions

A pregnant woman may have the same sicknesses as other people, such as:

- cough for more than a week
- high fever
- difficulty in breathing
- difficulty in passing urine.

All pregnant women with these conditions should be treated by a doctor. Delay in treatment may put both the baby's life and the mother's life in danger.

Drugs and medicines given to the mother also get into the baby's body. They may be too strong for the baby and may kill or harm it.

A pregnant woman should take medicines only when given by a doctor who knows that she is pregnant.

Bleeding from the genitals during pregnancy

Any bleeding from the genitals at any time in pregnancy means that something is wrong.

Bleeding before the baby has started to move in the womb

(1) If there is a little bleeding and no pain:

■ The woman must lie down and rest for 3 days or until there is no more bleeding.

■ If the bleeding does not stop after 3 days, arrange with the family to take her to the hospital.

■ Give her a bottle of rehydration fluid containing salt and sugar (like the one prepared for preventing dehydration in diarrhoea (see Unit 26)). She must drink one cup of this fluid every hour.

(2) If she has bleeding and there is pain, this means that the baby will probably come out and she may bleed a lot afterwards.

Make her lie down. Put a clean cloth over her genitals to catch the blood and anything else that comes out.

If the bleeding stops, make sure she stays in bed for 1 week. Tell the family she must not do heavy work or carry heavy things until after the baby starts to move strongly in her womb.

If the bleeding does not stop or it gets worse:

■ Make a bottle of rehydration fluid with salt, sugar and water (see Unit 26) and ask her to drink one cup of it every half hour.

■ Arrange with the family to take her to the hospital and to give her this drink as often as possible on the way.

Bleeding from the genitals after the baby has started to move in the womb

This is more serious. It means that the lives of both the baby and the mother are in danger. The baby will be born too soon or may die inside the mother. The mother may lose too much blood and may become very ill or die. She must go to the hospital immediately.

(1) If there is bleeding and no pain:

- Make her lie down and put a clean cloth over her genitals to catch the blood.

- Make a bottle of rehydration fluid (see Unit 26) and tell the family to make sure she drinks one cupful every half hour. Arrange with the family to take her to the nearest hospital. Go with them if you can and take with you any records you have made about her health.

(2) If there is bleeding and pain in the belly

- Find out what sort of pain it is. If the pain is coming and going regularly, she may be in labour. (See Unit 16 for instructions on how to help a woman in labour.) If the pain is there all the time and her belly is very painful when you touch it, this is dangerous. She must go to hospital *at once*.

- Give her a bottle of rehydration fluid and ask her to take one cupful every hour.

- Keep her warm and arrange for the family to carry her to the hospital.

- Go with her if you can and talk to the doctor yourself.

A pregnant woman with pain in her belly

If the pain comes and goes she is in labour. When a woman is in labour, the pain comes and goes at regular intervals. Sometimes it is a low back pain and sometimes a low front pain. It is never at the top of her belly.

If she has been pregnant for more than 8 months. Explain to the family that she may be in labour and that they should start to prepare for the delivery of the baby (see Unit 16).

If she has been pregnant for less than 8 months. You must advise her to rest completely to stop the pain so that the baby can stay inside her a little longer. Explain this to the family. Make her lie on her side in bed. She must not get up until she has had no pain for 1 whole day. She should have small meals 4 or 5 times a day. She must not do heavy work or lift heavy things when she gets up until after the baby is born. If the pain does not go away, she will probably deliver a small baby. You should be there to make sure the family knows how to care for it (see the section on small babies, Unit 17, on page 153).

Pain is there all the time. Feel the woman's belly. If it is hard and she tells you it is painful when you touch it, she should go to hospital at once. If the pain is not in the womb but somewhere else in the belly and the womb is not painful, then treat her for belly pain (see Unit 28).

A pregnant woman has swollen legs, hands, and face

This woman must go to hospital. Help the family arrange to take her to the hospital. Go with them, if you can, to explain the situation to the doctor. See also page 111.

A pregnant woman has fits or is unconscious

This woman is *very* ill and must go to the hospital *at once*. Explain to the family that this condition is very serious, and that to save her life she will need to go to hospital immediately after the fit.

To know what to do during a fit, see Unit 45. Give her *nothing* to eat. You may give her some water to drink.

What the family can do to improve the health of the pregnant woman in the family and protect her from illness

Pregnant women are often young. They usually do not make the decisions in the family. Therefore, you must get the cooperation of the whole family to improve and protect their health and the health of their babies. Every family wants to produce strong healthy babies. To do this, the mother must be strong and healthy too.

How to protect or improve the health of a pregnant woman

A pregnant woman should do less work than usual. Discuss with the family the work a pregnant woman does. If she is doing too much work, ask other family members to share some of her work.

Many young women start work very early in the morning and stop work only very late at night. Discuss with the family how other

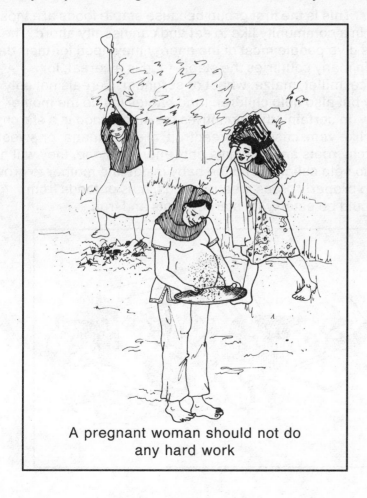

A pregnant woman should not do
any hard work

family members can do the early-morning and late-night work in order to give the pregnant woman more time to rest.

Many women carry heavy loads of water, fuel, animal feed, or crops every day. A pregnant woman must not carry heavy weights. Discuss with the family about who could do this work when the woman is pregnant.

Also, make sure that she gets a little more of each of the following groups of food each day.

Diet during pregnancy

Staple foods. This is the first group because staple foods are those that people in a community like to eat and can usually afford. The staple foods give people most of the energy they need for their day-to-day life. In many countries the staple food is a cereal; for example, rice, millet, maize, wheat or sorghum. Cereals not only give energy but also help children (and babies inside the mother's womb) grow. In certain other countries the staple food is a starchy root or fruit like yam, cassava, breadfruit, green banana, or sweet potato. Starchy roots and fruit give only energy. Alone, they will not be enough to help children and the baby inside the mother to grow and develop properly. Peas, beans, seeds, nuts or foods from animals should be eaten with starchy roots and fruit.

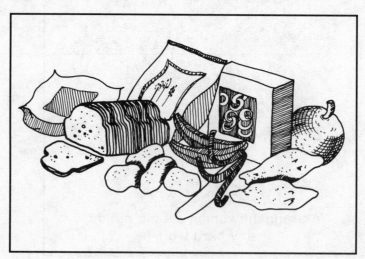

Peas, beans (legumes), seeds and nuts. These are important foods for growth. When eaten together with the staple food, they help children to grow well. They are also good for pregnant and breast-feeding women who must eat to help their babies grow strong. Some of these foods are: chick-peas, lentils, dal, soya beans, red beans, sesame seeds, melon seeds, groundnuts.

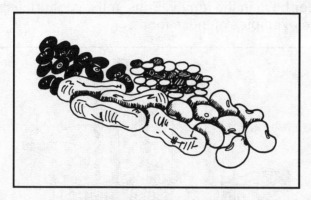

Dark green leafy and yellow vegetables. These vegetables are important for keeping the eyes healthy. They can also help make the blood strong. Children need these vegetables. So do women, especially those who are pregnant or breast-feeding. Some of these foods are: spinach, pak-choi cabbage, cassava leaves, many wild dark green leaves, carrot, pumpkin.

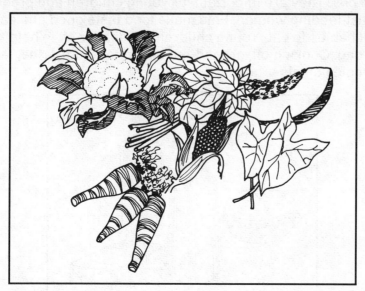

Foods from animals. Foods that come from animals help children
to grow and keep people strong and healthy. They are often
expensive. Whenever possible, small amounts of these foods
should be eaten with the staple food. Small children and women
who are breast-feeding or pregnant should have some of these
foods with the staple food. They need these foods more than the
men and older boys in the family. Eggs, milk, yoghurt, fish, poultry,
and meat are examples of these foods.

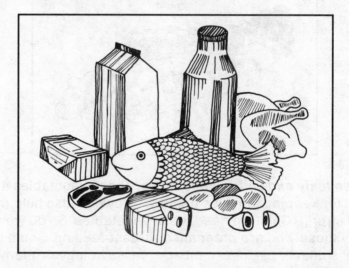

Fats and oils. They are important for young children and pregnant
and breast-feeding women. Fats make food taste good and easier
for small babies to eat. Young children need fat or oil to help them
grow strong. Cooking oil, ground-nut oil, butter, margarine, lard
are examples of this group.

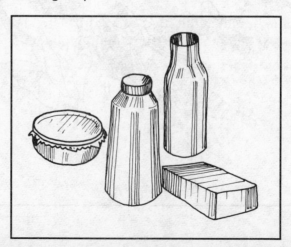

Fruit. Fruits are often not eaten as part of meals. They are useful in keeping the eyes and skin healthy. Fruit juices make good drinks for children, pregnant women, and women who are taking iron pills. They help the body to use the iron. Pawpaw (papaya), mango, orange, limes, cashew fruit, guava, pineapple, and soursop are examples from this food group.

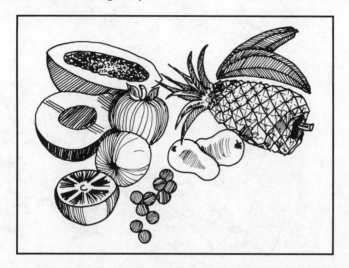

Discuss with the family what meals they make, what other foods they can get locally, and how these may be used to improve the diet of a pregnant woman.

How to protect pregnant women from illness

Every pregnant woman should visit the health centre in early pregnancy because:

■ It is only at the health centre that she can get an injection that will prevent her and her baby from getting tetanus.

■ The health centre staff will help the family to decide which is the safest place for her baby to be born.

■ The health centre staff can make checks on the health of the mother and the unborn baby (which cannot be done in the village).

Discuss the reasons with the family. Arrange with them a time to visit the health centre when it is convenient for the family *and* the health centre.

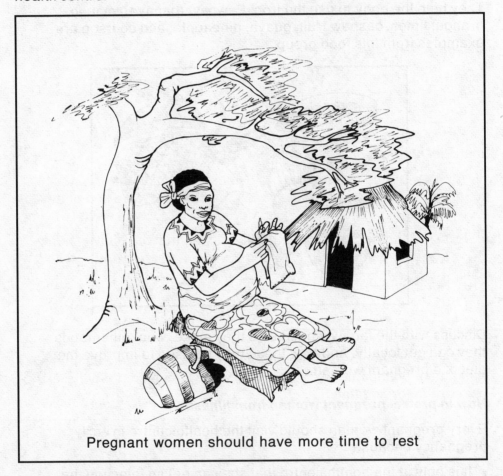

Pregnant women should have more time to rest

How to prepare for the birth of the baby

Help the family to make the right decisions about the following questions:

- Which is the safest place for the birth of the baby (home, health centre, or hospital)?
- If the baby is to be born at home, who will help with the delivery of the baby (midwife, nurse, CHW)?

- What things will be needed for the delivery?

- How will the baby be clothed and kept warm?

- If the baby is to be born at the health centre or hospital, when should the woman go there?

- Who will go with her?

- How will she get there and get back again?

- What will she need to take with her?

If the baby is to be born at home, help the family to prepare the material needed for a safe delivery

The family should get several old pieces of cloth or sacking, wash them well with soap and water, and then dry them on a line or a tree in the sun but *not* on the ground. These cloths will be used:

- To spread under the mother at delivery so that the baby is born on to a safe place

- To wrap the new baby in

- To put over the vulva to catch blood loss for as long as needed after the delivery.

Cut four strips of cloth 20 cm long and 6–7 cm wide and boil them; hang them on the line to dry in the hot sun. These are for tying the cord before cutting it.

Get a *new* razor blade and keep it ready without opening the packet.

Wrap all these items in *one* of the clean cloths. Tie it safely and put it in a safe clean place where it cannot be touched until needed for delivery.

Community action for keeping pregnant women healthy

(1) Meet with the community to discuss what they remember about problems related to births. For example:

- babies born too early

■ mothers who had severe bleeding

■ mothers who died or who were very ill

■ babies who were born dead or died soon after birth.

(2) Discuss with them what happens in a family when a mother becomes very ill or dies.

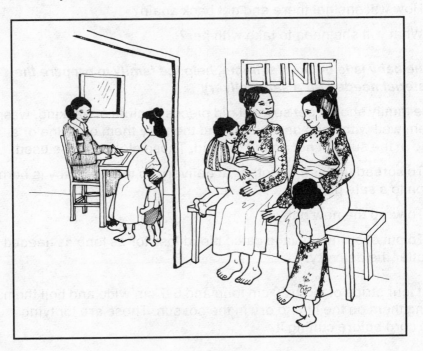

(3) Explain that most of the problems can be prevented by following the simple rules given below.

■ Pregnancy should be prevented until the woman is old enough and healthy enough to have a baby safely.

■ Every pregnant woman should be examined by trained health staff at the nearest clinic or health centre as early in pregnancy as possible.

■ Every pregnant woman should get 1 or 2 injections during pregnancy to prevent tetanus.

■ The delivery should take place in the safest possible place. The place should be carefully chosen, considering the state of health of the pregnant woman.

■ The person who is to help with the birth should be trained to do so. She should wash her hands carefully before delivery, and use only clean equipment.

(4) Discuss with the community how they can make sure that the above rules are followed in the whole community.

(5) Meet with the women's groups and help them to decide what they can do to:

■ encourage families to provide extra food and rest for pregnant women

■ provide extra food for very thin pregnant women

■ make sure that someone goes with the women to the health centre for immunization and for care when needed

■ make sure that traditional birth attendants receive some training to make their care safer

■ learn about safe practices during delivery and insist that these are followed

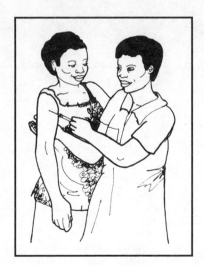

■ help you to identify all pregnant women in the community so that you can visit them and talk to their families.

The collection and use of information in pregnancy

You should write down information about pregnant women to help you to:

■ plan your work and make more visits to those who most need your help

■ remember what the family has agreed to do as a result of your discussions; you can then check if it has been done

■ identify problems that can be solved by group action in the community, for example, helping pregnant women in their daily tasks

■ identify problems that must be solved with the help of the health service staff

■ share information with the health team.

See also Units 51 and 52.

Unit 16

Labour and delivery

When the baby is ready to live outside the mother's body, the womb begins to press the baby out. This is called labour. It ends when the baby and the afterbirth (placenta) are outside the mother's body.

Most labours and deliveries are normal but, to deal with any difficulties that may arise, a trained person should attend all deliveries. You must make sure therefore that the family arranges for such a trained attendant.

All births must be recorded and reported as soon as possible, according to the instructions you receive in your country or district.

Learning objectives

After studying this unit you should be able to:

1 Explain to families how the baby comes out of the mother's body, and what care they should take during delivery.

2 Decide whether a woman is in labour.

3 Prepare, with the help of the family, everything needed for a safe delivery.

4 Help at the time of delivery, using the materials prepared earlier.

5 Decide the right moment when a mother should be sent to the nearest hospital; arrange this journey with the family and arrange for care to be given during the journey.

6 Take emergency action:

- if some other part of the baby except the top of the head comes first

- if more than a little blood runs from the mother's opening after the baby is born

- if the placenta (afterbirth) does not come out within half an hour of birth.

7 Discuss with community leaders and families community action to improve the health of expectant mothers and to prevent serious illness or death.

How the baby is born

The baby and the **placenta** are in a bag of water inside the mother's womb. The baby is connected to the placenta by the umbilical cord. When the womb starts to open, the mother will have regular pains which come faster and faster as the opening gets wider. This opening is inside the mother and you cannot see it. Opening of the womb takes about 12 hours in the first pregnancy but usually a much shorter time in later pregnancies. Give the mother small drinks of a water and sugar mixture during labour.

When the womb is fully open, the bag of water will burst and the baby will slide down inside the mother. When this happens, the mother will want to push the baby out. When she starts to push, the delivery is near and she should be in the clean place prepared for the delivery.

You will soon be able to see the baby at the **vulva**. With every push, the baby will come out a bit more. Tell the mother not to hurry. She will need to rest after each push.

The baby's head will come out slowly, and then the shoulders and the rest of the baby will follow quickly. The baby will still be attached to the placenta by the cord. You will have to tie and then cut the cord. About 10 minutes after the baby is born, the womb will become small and push out the placenta and the bag that held the water. At this time the mother may bleed about a cupful of blood; this is normal.

Within one or two minutes of being born, the baby will take his first breath and may cry. After that you should put the baby to the mother's breast and let the baby suck. This feed is very good for the baby, and the baby's sucking causes the womb to become hard and this stops the bleeding.

When the baby has had the feed, the mother will be hungry and thirsty. Give her sweet food and drink. Then let her and the baby rest.

How to know if a woman is in labour

A woman is in labour when:

- The pain comes regularly every 10 minutes or more often. The woman feels this pain at the bottom of her back or at the bottom of her belly. With each pain, the top of her womb feels hard.

- A sticky jelly mixed with blood comes out of her vagina.

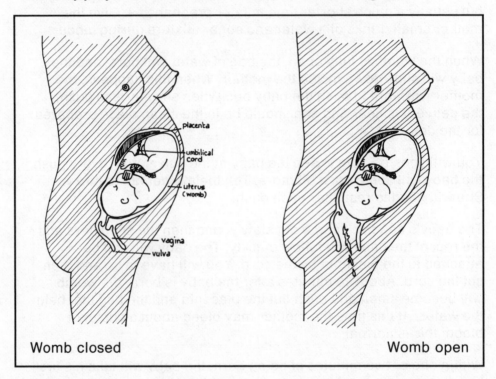

placenta

umbilical cord

uterus (womb)

vagina

vulva

Womb closed   Womb open

To find out whether she is in labour:

- Ask the pregnant woman or the women who are with her whether she is having regular pains.

- Put your hand gently on the top of her belly to feel whether it goes hard with the pain.

Prepare everything needed for a safe delivery

When you are sure that the mother is in labour, prepare for delivery as follows:

- Tell the mother that she must be patient: labour takes time.

- She must not try to push the baby out until she feels the urge to do so. Her body will tell her when it is time to push the baby out.

- Ask all the people who can be of no help to leave the room. The mother should choose whom she would like to stay.

- Ask the mother to pass urine and faeces if she can. Someone should go with her to help her.

- Afterwards ask her to wash her hands carefully with soap and clean water. She should then wash her genitals, and then her legs and feet.

- She should then put on clean clothes. The woman is now ready for the delivery.

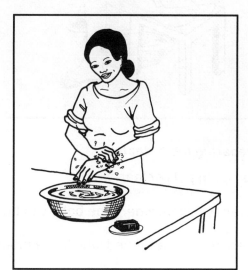

Preparing for delivery

1. Pass urine and faeces.
2. Wash hands with soap and water.

3. Wash the genitals.

4. Wash the legs and feet.

5. Put on clean clothes.

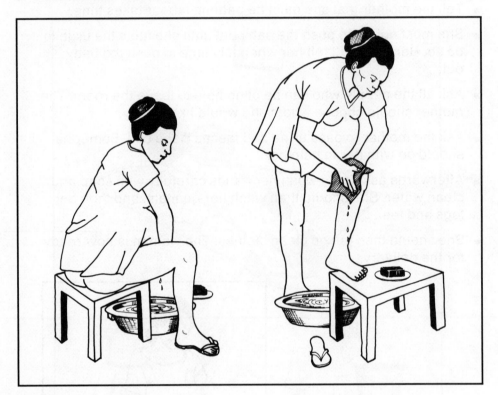

Preparing the birthplace

Boil a big pot of clean water.

Clean the room where the baby will be born.

Prepare the mat or bed where the mother will give birth.

Ask the family for the package of material they prepared for delivery (see Unit 15). If they did not make a package ask them to find clean cloths that you can use. Tear four strips of the cloth and put them into the water to boil. Ask for an *unused* razor blade.

Scrub one basin very well. When the water has boiled, put some of it in the basin to cool. Keep the rest on the fire to boil until only half is left; then take it off the fire to cool. Keep it covered until it is needed.

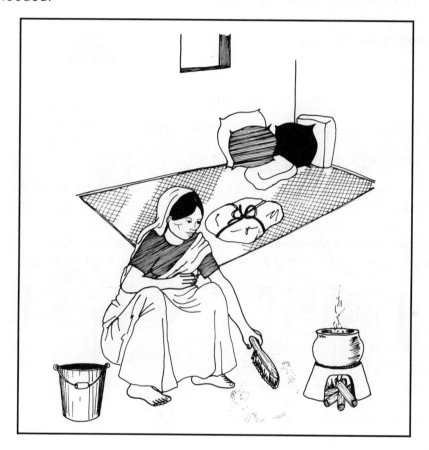

Prepare yourself to help

Your fingernails should be short and clean.

Roll up your sleeves. With soap and a scrubbing brush, scrub your hands, nails and arms to the elbow, if possible under running water.

Put a bowl of water and the soap close to where the mother will give birth. You may need to wash your hands many times.

Now you are ready to help with the delivery.

Helping at the delivery

The delivery

The baby will be born very soon when:

- the pains come quickly (every 2–3 minutes)
- the mother feels the urge to push
- with every pain you can see a little of the baby appearing at the vulva.

Wash your hands again very carefully. Then lay a large clean cloth (the one prepared earlier) on the mat or bed prepared for birth.

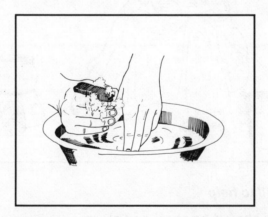

There are several positions in which a woman can deliver. The person attending the delivery (nurse, midwife, or CHW) should help the woman decide which one is the most comfortable for her.

Ask the woman to place herself on the mat in the position that she has selected for delivery (kneeling, sitting, squatting, lying).

Every time the mother has a pain, ask her to push hard. When she has no pain she must *not* push.

When the baby's head is out, wipe its nose and mouth with a clean cloth. Feel round the neck for the cord; it feels like a soft rope. If you feel it, try to draw it gently over the baby's head.

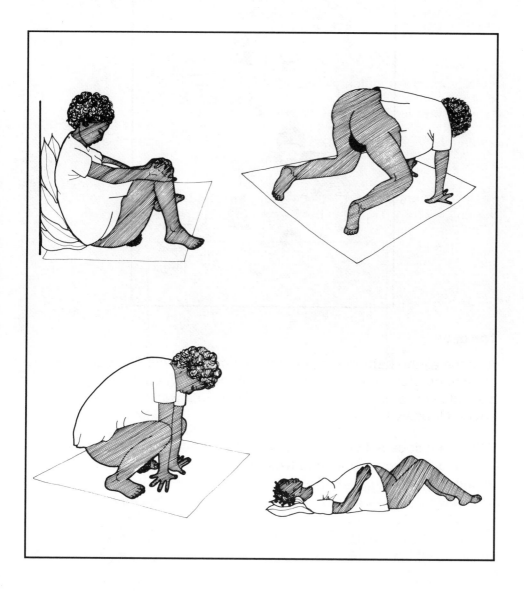

The mother's body must be *very* close to the mat so that the baby will not drop but slide out on to the prepared mat.

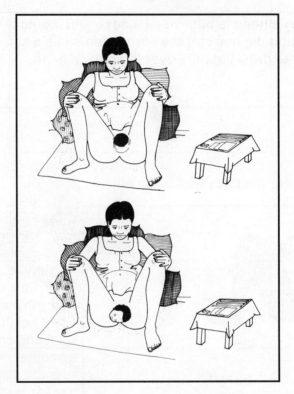

The baby

As soon as the baby comes out hold it upside down. The baby will cry immediately or within one or two minutes. When the baby has started to breathe normally, dry it softly with a warm, dry cloth and cover it loosely to keep it warm.

If the baby does not cry within one or two minutes, you may have to help it to do so by giving mouth-to-mouth resuscitation (see Annex 2, page 397).

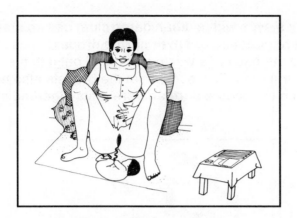

What to do after the baby has come out

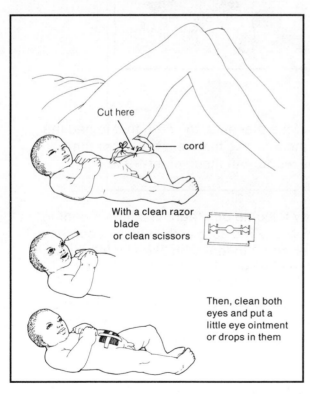

Cut here

cord

With a clean razor
blade
or clean scissors

Then, clean both
eyes and put a
little eye ointment
or drops in them

Take one of the strips of cloth or string from the package and tie it tightly round the cord, one little finger's length away from the belly of the baby. Tie a second one tightly another little finger's length away. Take the razor blade from the package and cut *between* the two knots (see picture).

Wipe the baby's eyes with a clean damp cloth or swab, and put tetracycline eye ointment or silver nitrate drops into each eye (see Unit 37). Wrap the baby in a warm cloth, and put it to the mother's breast for its first feed. This sucking at the breasts also helps the mother's womb to become hard and prevents bleeding after delivery.

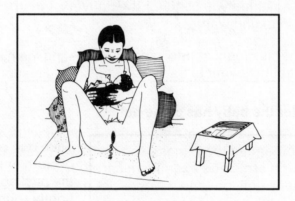

The afterbirth (*placenta*)

The afterbirth is made up of the placenta, the cord that joined the placenta to the baby, and the thin bag that held the water that surrounded the baby in the womb. All these must come out together.

When the afterbirth is ready to come out, there is a little bleeding from the vagina (about a cupful). The cord at the vulva becomes a little longer, and the mother starts to feel pain like she felt during labour, but the pain is not so intense.

Ask the mother to push or to cough, and the afterbirth will come out easily. *Do not pull on the cord.* Let the family dispose of the afterbirth in the customary way, by burning or burying, for example.

Clean the mother, the material and the house

When the baby is born and the afterbirth has been put away, the mother should be cleaned, made comfortable, and allowed to rest.

Wash the blood from the mother's body with the boiled water that is left. When she is clean, cover her genitals with one of the clean cloths from the package. The wet and blood-stained cloths should be removed from the mother's bed. The area around the bed should also be cleaned.

Wash and boil anything you used for the delivery. Wash your hands carefully with soap and water.

When the mother is clean, comfortable, and resting, give her a drink and something sweet to eat. Then she should sleep.

Examining the baby and dressing the cord

After the baby has had his first feed and has rested while you cleaned the mother and the things used in delivery, take the baby from the mother's arms and examine it carefully. Wash it quickly with warm water or oil, or wipe it with a clean cloth, according to custom. Do not let the baby get cold. Show the family how to dress the cord if the dressing gets dirty:

- First wash your hands with soap and water.

- Then take a small piece of cloth and put it over the cut end of the cord. Tie it to the bottom of the cord and keep it covered (see drawings).

- Another way of dressing the cord is to lay the cord flat on the baby's belly, with the cut end towards the baby's head, and to wrap a small strip of **clean** cloth like a bandage loosely round the baby's body to keep the cord from getting wet with urine.

Tell the family and repeat very firmly that they should only touch the cord after washing their hands with soap and water. Also, only clean cloths (washed with soap and water and dried on a line or tree in the hot sun) should be used for dressing the cord and collecting and wiping blood off the mother's vulva. **No powder or mud or dung or anything else must be put on or near the cord.**

How to dress the cord

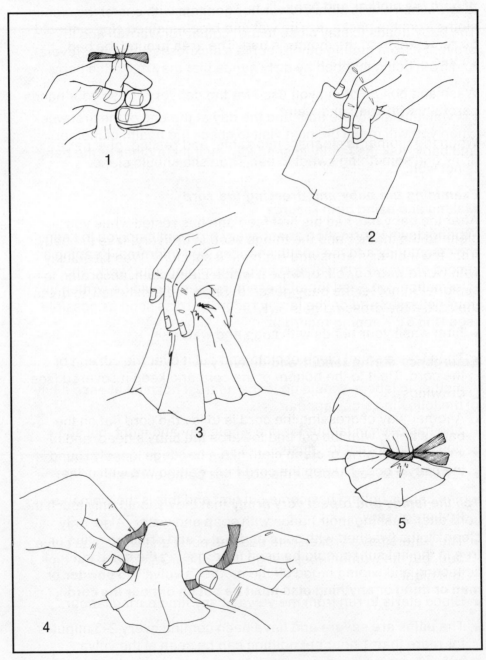

Remind the family of the importance of breast-feeding for the health of both the mother and baby.

The baby needs to stay close to the mother for warmth and to prevent it from getting other people's sicknesses (coughs, fevers), and from being touched by dirty hands that may make the baby sick.

Fix with the family the time and the day at the end of the first week when you will make the next visit to check the health of mother and baby. Ask the family to send for you if the mother or the baby is not well.

Making and using birth records

Writing down information about every birth will help you to keep the community and the health services well informed. Keeping a record of every birth will also help you to plan your work. The information you need for all these purposes should be written in your notebook and on the family record card as soon as possible (see Unit 51: Keeping records).

Emergency during labour and delivery

A mother in labour should go to the nearest hospital **at once** if any of the following signs appear:

- She has been in labour for one whole day and night, but she does not yet want to "push".

- A hand, arm, leg, foot, or the cord has come out first.

- The baby's bottom has come out first and this is the woman's first pregnancy.

- The waters have broken (the bag has burst and water has come out), but the woman does not go into labour within one full day and night.

- Blood starts to run from the vulva at any time during labour.

- The pains are severe and have been coming every 2–3 minutes for more than 1 hour but nothing can be seen at the vulva.

- The mother is pushing and the part of the baby you can see at the opening does not come out any further in 1 hour.

- The mother has pain all over her belly and the belly is very painful to touch.

- The mother has fits or becomes unconscious.

How to take her to the hospital

During the journey to the hospital:

- The mother should be carried lying down, if possible

- Take one or two bottles of rehydration fluid (water with salt and sugar) and a cup, and let the woman drink as often as possible during the journey

- Keep the woman warm

- Go with the woman and take with you the prepared package for delivery, in case she has the baby on the way to the hospital.

Emergency care

If the baby's bottom comes out first and it is not possible to take the woman to hospital

Do not touch the baby. The baby will be easily born till the shoulders come out. The baby's belly must be facing towards the floor. If it is not, then cover the baby with a warm clean cloth and gently and slowly turn it so that you can see its back.

When its chest shows you that it is beginning to breathe, lift it up gently by the feet, with the body at full stretch, till it is upside down.

You should now be able to see its mouth and nose at the vulva. Clean the mouth and nose with a clean cloth so that the baby can breathe air. Ask the mother to push gently, and the head will come out.

If the mother bleeds after the birth of the baby and the afterbirth is still inside

Put the baby to the breast and help it to suck. If the baby is too weak to suck, ask one of the women present to gently pull the mother's nipple just like a baby would pull the nipple if it were sucking.

Put your hand on the mother's belly just below the navel. You should feel a soft lump. Rub this gently and quickly with your fingers until it becomes hard. The bleeding will stop. Repeat this every time the lump becomes soft until you see that the cord is getting longer.

The next time the uterus gets hard after the cord has lengthened, ask the mother to push, and the afterbirth should come out.

If the mother bleeds after the afterbirth has come out

Give her one tablet of ergometrine 0.2 mg; if necessary, this dose may be repeated once or twice (see Annex 1).

Put the baby to the breast and try to make it suck. If it cannot suck, ask one of the women in the room to gently pull the mother's nipple just like a baby would pull the nipple if it were sucking.

Find the top of the womb by putting your hand on the mother's belly below the navel. It will feel like a soft ball. Rub it gently but quickly with your fingers till it becomes hard. This might take some time.

Ask another woman in the room to make a hot sweet drink for the mother and to cover her with a blanket. When the bleeding stops, put the mother's hand on the hard womb and tell her to rub it every time she feels blood running out. *The womb must stay hard.*

If the bleeding does not stop she must be carried to a hospital or the nearest health centre *at once*, with the baby.

Before the journey, put as many clean cloths as possible over her vulva to collect all the blood, and ask the women to prepare one

143

or two bottles of rehydration fluid (water with salt and sugar) to take with you. On the way give the mother drinks of rehydration fluid and try to keep the womb hard.

If the afterbirth does not come out within half an hour of birth

Give the mother a drink and ask her to try to pass urine. After that check if the womb is hard. Ask her to cough forcefully once or twice. The afterbirth should drop out.

If it does not drop out, *do not pull the cord*. If the placenta is stuck firmly to the inside of the womb, you *cannot* pull it off. If you pull, you may pull out the womb too. This is *very dangerous* and could kill the mother. Take her to the nearest hospital or health centre as soon as possible, keeping her warm and giving her drinks on the way.

Discussions with the community

First, review carefully Units 15 and 16.

The community can help to improve the health of women and babies. Discuss with the various community groups and families:

(1) Why the health of the mother in the family is important.

(2) How pregnancy begins and how the baby grows inside the mother; what the mother needs to make the baby strong and healthy; what happens if the mother works too hard or gets too little food or rest.

(3) What are the risk factors in pregnancy; when it is less safe to have a baby; which pregnant women need *extra* care; what is the danger to the mother and baby if a woman who has any of the risk factors gives birth at home.

(4) How to tell when a pregnant woman needs to be seen urgently by a midwife or doctor; which women should have their babies in the clinic or hospital.

(5) Why women must be immunized against tetanus.

(6) Why cleanliness is important at the time of delivery and how

the proper care of the cord prevents tetanus of the newborn child; why it is important to prepare a "delivery package" during pregnancy and to store it safely and not open it until delivery.

At delivery the family must insist that the midwife:

- scrubs her hands with soap and water
- uses cloths from the prepared package to prepare the delivery mat
- uses a *new* razor blade to cut the cord
- puts a clean cloth on the baby's cut cord and *nothing else*.

(7) What the community can do to help a family to take a pregnant woman to hospital immediately.

(8) If the woman needs to be carried, how this can be done.

(9) Which is the quickest way to hospital?

(10) Who will help to carry the woman?

(11) If extra money is needed, can the community help? How?

(12) What must a family do to get this help?

(13) How can *all* families know that such help is available?

Unit 17

First few weeks after delivery

After the baby is born, many changes take place in the woman's body. The womb must get small again. The mother's breasts must start making enough milk for the baby. For all this, the mother's body needs special care.

The baby also needs a lot of care.

Learning objectives

After studying this unit you should be able to:

1 Obtain information about a recent birth from the mother, family, or birth attendant, and record it or report it to the health centre.

2 Put questions to and examine a woman who gave birth in the previous week.

3 List the common problems of mothers after childbirth and discuss with the family how they can manage them.

4 Examine a newly born baby and question the family about the care being given to the baby.

5 Explain to mothers the common problems of newborn babies and how to manage them.

6 Discuss with the family members what they can do to keep the mother and baby healthy.

7 Keep the community informed about health problems of mothers and newborn babies, and get the community's cooperation in solving them.

Obtaining information about recent births

When you attend a birth you have the information you need. When someone else (e.g., the TBA) attends, you must get information from that person or from the family, as soon as possible. *Visit the house where the birth took place.*

The information you need is:

- How is the mother? What is her name?
- How is the baby?
- Who attended the delivery?
- Were there any difficulties during labour?
- Did the midwife wash her hands before the delivery?
- What was used to cut and dress the cord?

If either the mother or the baby has died it may be easier to talk to the birth attendant or another person who was present at the delivery rather than to members of the family.

Write down all the information you can get in your notebook and fill in your *birth-records book* (see Unit 51).

How to talk to and examine the mother

First, find out how she is feeling. Let her talk first before you ask questions. Then ask her whether she is:

- sleeping well
- eating two good meals a day, with a little snack between meals
- passing urine normally (after childbirth a woman passes a lot of urine)
- drinking plenty of fluids (fluids will help her to make enough milk for the baby)
- walking around the house when she likes to, walking to the toilet to wash herself
- using clean water to wash her breasts and genitals every day.

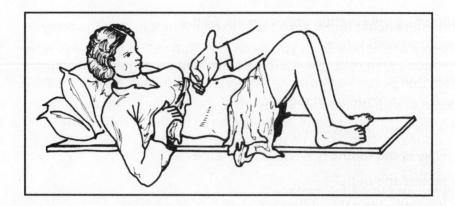

Examine her to make sure that her womb is becoming small again.

Explain to her what you are doing. If you have a thermometer, use it to find out if she has fever. If you do not have a thermometer, feel her forehead with your hand. If it is hot, she has fever.

Put your hand on the lower part of the belly and press gently. You will feel something hard and round. This is the womb. Make her also feel this. Tell her that if she bleeds she should rub it gently and the bleeding will stop.

Common problems of the mother in the first few weeks after birth

A breast feels hard and hot

The mother complains that her breasts feel heavy and painful. Ask the family to get a bowl of hot water and a bowl of cold water, and two clean cloths. Show the family how to bathe the breasts, first with cold water and then with hot water. Gently squeeze out a little milk from one breast till the brown part around the nipple is soft. Put the baby to that breast. Do the same with the other breast. Explain to the family that the baby should feed often, and that while the breasts are hard the mother should press out a little milk before letting the baby suck. Give her 2 aspirins to ease the pain.

Sore nipples

Advise the mother to wash and dry the nipples carefully after each feed. When they are dry, she should rub on some oil to keep them soft. She should make sure that the entire nipple is in the baby's mouth when it feeds.

After-pains

These are pains like labour pains in the bottom of the belly. They are usually more severe when the baby feeds. They usually disappear within a few days. Ask the family to give the mother 2 aspirins if the pains are bad.

Crying and unhappy mother

Sometimes the mother feels sad and weak, and she may cry and may not be able to sleep well. She may also behave abnormally. Explain to the family that they must be patient with her and that she will probably improve in a few days. If she does not feel better after a few days, she should see a doctor at the health centre or hospital.

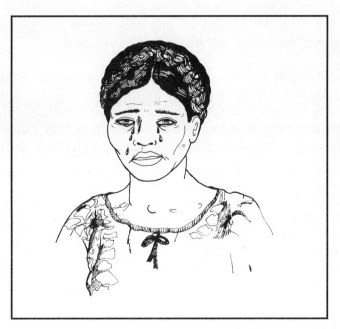

Problems for which a mother must go the hospital or health centre

You should send the mother to the nearest health centre or hospital if:

- She has fever for more than 2 days.

- The blood coming out of her genitals smells bad or is bright red.

- She has so much pain in the breast that she cannot feed the baby.

- One of her legs is swollen and painful to touch. She will probably also have a fever. She should rest and not walk.

- She becomes very sad and cries a lot and cannot sleep well.

Bleeding from the genitals

It is normal for a mother to lose a little blood during the first few days after the birth. The blood usually gets darker and becomes less during the first week; it then becomes yellowish.

If at any time *bright red* blood runs out, there is something wrong. You must take her to the hospital or health centre. Put a bowl or clean cloth by her genitals to collect any blood that runs out. Press gently her lower belly and locate the womb. Rub it till it goes hard. This will make more blood come at first, but soon the bleeding will stop.

Tell the family to make hot sweet drinks for her. Wipe the blood from her genitals and legs, dress her in clean clothes, and take her quickly to the hospital or health centre. Give her plenty of rehydration fluid to drink on the way and tell the doctor or midwife how much blood she has lost. If the mother goes to the hospital, the baby should go too, so that breast-feeding can continue.

How to examine the baby

First talk to the mother, and, if possible, also the father. Ask the mother the following questions.

- Is the baby feeding from *both* breasts every time it wants to feed? If not, suggest that this be done.

- Does the baby stay close to the mother so that it keeps warm and does not get passed from person to person? People who have any illness should not go near the baby.

- Is the baby passing urine normally?

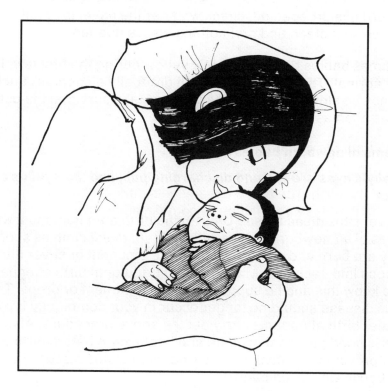

- Is the baby passing faeces normally? During the first few days after birth the faeces will be blackish. This is normal. Later, they will turn brown, and finally yellow.

Now examine the baby. First, wash your hands. Take off the baby's clothes. Remember that the baby is very small and that too many clothes make it hard for it to breathe properly. Explain this to the family.

If you have weighing scales, weigh the baby. If not, try to decide whether it is normal in size and weight (see Unit 20).

The cord should have only a clean cloth covering it. If there is any mud or ash or anything else on the cord, explain to the family how dangerous this is and suggest that they wash it off and put on a clean dressing.

If the cord has dropped off, check whether the navel is dry. It should be kept clean and dry; nothing else is needed.

Sometimes babies become slightly yellow during the first few days. This is normal. The yellow colour will gradually disappear. Such a baby may be slow to feed for a few days. Make sure that the baby is fed as often as it wants to feed.

Problems of newborn babies

The baby's eyes are red and discharging pus, and the eyelids are swollen

To prevent this disease (see Unit 16) the birth attendant must wipe the eyes of *all* newborn babies with a clean, moist cloth as soon as they are born and put tetracycline eye ointment or silver nitrate eye drops into each eye. Midwives and traditional birth attendants should know this and be supplied with the ointment or drops. This serious disease should no longer occur in your community if you and other birth attendants carry out the above procedure. Also, mother's good personal hygiene and health care before birth will help to prevent this infection. The treatment of this disease is described in Unit 37 on page 287.

The baby cries a lot

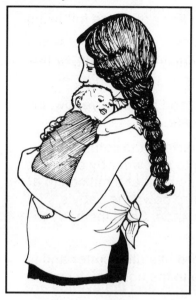

(1) The baby has probably swallowed air during feeding. Show the mother how to hold the baby against her shoulder and gently pat its back after each feed (see picture). Once the air comes up from the stomach, the baby will feel better.

(2) The baby may be too hot and sweating. Take off some of the clothes. The mother should give it a feed to put back some of the water lost in sweating. Warn the family about too many clothes and coverings.

The baby is very small (less than 2500 g)

If the baby was born about the right time, it will feel hungry normally and will feed well. The baby should be put to the breast as often as it wants to feed. Make sure the family knows that the mother must have extra food and drinks. The baby should sleep between feeds; this helps it to use the milk and to grow quickly.

If the baby was born more than one month too early, it may not live without special care. The family must decide about the care. They can take it to hospital (the mother must also go to feed it). If they want to keep the baby at home and if the baby is too weak to suck at the mother's breast, ask the mother to squeeze milk out from her breasts and feed it to the baby with a clean *boiled* spoon. Without milk the baby will not grow. The baby must be kept warm and clean, and should be picked up as little as possible.

Problems for which the baby must be taken to the hospital

Take the baby quickly to the hospital if you find any of the following problems:

(1) *Abnormal breathing.* The breathing is noisy and difficult, or the baby's belly is sucked in with each breath.

(2) *Yellowness.* The baby is yellow at birth and remains yellow, or starts to go yellow after the first 10 days of life.

(3) *The baby has high fever.* If there is malaria in the community, take *half* a tablet of **chloroquine**, crush it into a powder by pressing it between two spoons, squeeze some of the mother's milk on to a spoon with the powder, and pour the mixture down the baby's throat, with the baby lying on the mother's knee. Send the baby to the health centre or hospital as soon as possible.

Ask what was used to dress and cut the cord. If a dirty cutter and dressing were used, take the baby *at once* to the hospital. It cannot be treated at home.

(4) *The baby has a fit, goes stiff and cannot open his mouth.* This is probably **tetanus**. The baby should go to the hospital *at once*.

Remember!

If the baby must go to the hospital, the mother must also go to feed the baby. Breast-feeding should not stop.

Discussions with the family

Each family is different. When you give them advice you must try to give it in a friendly way so that they are glad to accept and follow your suggestions.

Advice for the mother

After a delivery a mother needs:

(1) more food and drink than usual

(2) more rest and sleep than usual

(3) to keep very clean

(4) to prevent pregnancy for the next two years (see Unit 18).

Discuss with the woman and her husband the reasons for not becoming pregnant for 2 years. Use the arguments given in Unit 18.

Remind them that frequent breast-feeding can help to prevent pregnancy for 3–4 months. After that she or her husband will need to take special steps to prevent pregnancy.

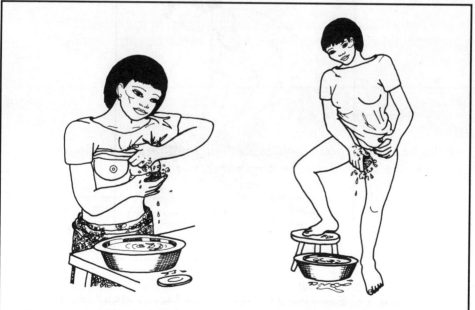

Every day the mother should wash her whole body including her breasts and her genitals with soap and water

The mother must stay close to the baby. Only the mother can provide the right food for the baby. Wherever the mother goes, the baby should go with her.

What the baby needs after birth

(1) *Breast-feeding*. The thick, yellow milk of the first 2–3 days after delivery (colostrum) is very important for the baby. White milk will come easier if the baby feeds from the breast *often* from the moment of birth. Breast milk is both food and drink; the baby needs nothing else till the age of four months.

(2) *Warmth*. The mother should remain close to the baby.

(3) *To be kept clean*. The mother should know how to bath the baby.

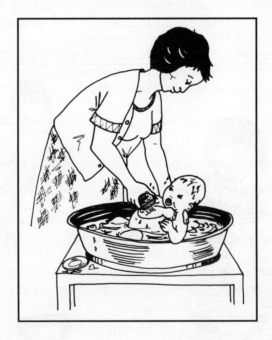

(4) *Immunization*. See Unit 21. Remind the family about childhood illnesses: tuberculosis (TB), whooping cough, diphtheria, tetanus, measles, poliomyelitis. Arrange with the family when and where to go to get immunizations against these diseases.

(5) *To be loved and cuddled.* A baby needs a lot of love and attention. Encourage the family to talk to the baby. Babies learn things faster when parents talk to them.

Getting the community's support

Families will do what you advise them to do if the whole community agrees with your advice.

Discuss with the community what can be done to make sure that in every family:

- the mother can have extra food and drink, take more rest and do less work than usual
- the baby is made to suck at the breasts of the mother in the first hour after birth
- the baby's cord is kept very clean
- *all* babies receive *all* the immunizations so that no child will catch or die from measles, whooping cough, diphtheria, tetanus, poliomyelitis or tuberculosis (see Unit 21).

Discuss with the community what can be done about problems such as:

- deaths of mothers in childbirth, and deaths of newborn babies
- sending mothers and new babies to hospital in emergencies
- people refusing immunizations for their babies
- people refusing help with child-spacing.

Discuss with the community why these problems occur and what the community or the health workers can do to prevent them in the future.

Planning a family

---

*Planning a family means having children when the family
wants to and can afford to have them.*

*Family planning can help avoid some of the risk factors of
pregnancy (see Unit 15). There are several simple and
reliable methods available for preventing pregnancies.*

Learning objectives

After studying this unit you should be able to:

1 Give information to families and the community to help them to
  think about planning their families.

2 Give simple explanations about the methods of family planning
  they can use.

3 Treat simple problems related to the use of family planning
  methods and know when to send a person or a couple to the
  health centre.

4 Keep records and follow up couples using a method of family
  planning.

5 Identify couples who have no children but would like to have a
  child, and give them information.

Information to help people to think about planning their families

For the family

After 17 years of age a woman's body is fully grown. Pregnancy after this age produces bigger, healthier babies than if it occurs at a younger age.

A baby's health will suffer if it is not allowed to continue breast-feeding because the mother is pregnant again too soon after the birth. Mothers' bodies need a long time, sometimes 2 years or more, to get back to full strength after the birth of a baby.

A mother who is sick should complete the treatment and get well before starting a pregnancy.

If there are risk factors, the woman should avoid becoming pregnant (see Unit 15).

For community groups

Information given to the family must also be given to community groups. People who decide to plan and space their families in order to improve family health often need the support of others.

It is the task of community leaders to arrange things so that everyone can be well.

To help community leaders to think about family planning it is useful to ask questions and to let them discuss the possible answers. Such questions might be:

(1) What can we do to make sure that every pregnancy ends in a strong healthy baby and a strong healthy mother?

(2) What is the best age to have a baby?

(3) Is it good to have a baby every year?

For those who want to space their children or want to have no more children

The following are simple explanations that you can give to a couple who want information before making a decision about which

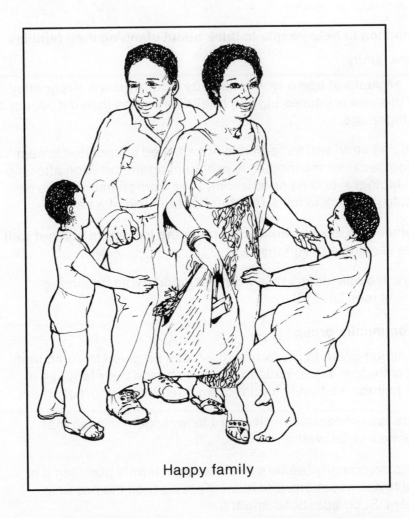

Happy family

method to choose. Not all the methods described here may be available in your area. Find out which of the methods are available. Then mark them on your book and tell people about them. Do *not* discuss other methods.

All methods described in section 1 below can be stopped at once if the family decides to have another child.

When a couple decide on a method from section 2 below, they will not be able to have any more children.

Use the diagrams in this book to explain the methods to families.

(1) *Family planning methods that can be stopped when the family wants to have a child*

The condom

This is a rubber cover that is rolled over the hard penis just before intercourse. It stops the man's sperm from getting to the woman's egg. Condoms are easy to use and easy to get. In our community we can get them from:

....

(write here from where the couple can get them)

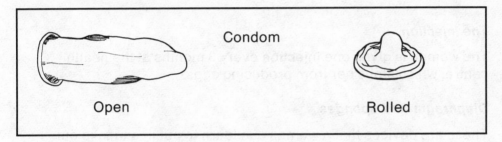

Condom

Open   Rolled

The pill

A little tablet is taken by the mother *every* day. This stops her body from making eggs. It is not good for every woman. The health staff at the clinic will do some tests to decide which women cannot take it.

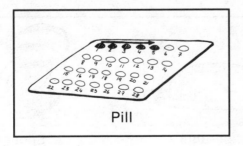

Pill

The loop (intrauterine device—IUD)

This is a device that is put
inside the woman's womb. It
makes it difficult for the egg to
stay there and grow into a
baby. The woman must go to
the health centre to have it put
inside her.

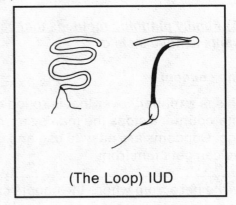

(The Loop) IUD

The injection

The woman is given one injection every 3 months at the health
centre, which stops her from producing eggs.

Diaphragm and sponges

These are devices that a woman can learn to put in and take out
herself. They stop the man's sperm from getting to the woman's
egg. Diaphragms are usually used with a jelly, and can be washed
and used more than once. The correct size of diaphragm needs to
be used so the woman will have to go to the health centre where
the staff can select the right one. Sponges, on the other hand, are
used only once, and then thrown away. One size is suitable for all
women.

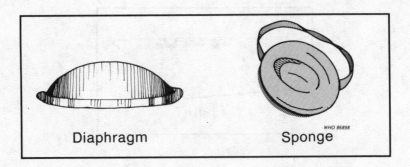

Diaphragm   Sponge

Natural methods

To use these, the woman and the man must know when the woman's body is producing an egg. Around this time they must *not* have sexual relations if they want to avoid pregnancy. They should visit the health centre to learn how to use these methods. For some couples they are easy to use. Remember, these methods do not always work. Even when using them the woman may become pregnant.

Withdrawal or "pull-out" method

The man takes his penis out of the woman's body before his sperm starts to come out of his body. It may be difficult to do this safely and it may not give full sexual satisfaction to both partners.

Home methods

Many communities have their own traditional methods of preventing pregnancy. Some are dangerous and some are useless. Ask your health centre staff about them. Some of the home methods may be of help until the time when a couple can go to the health centre for advice. One such method is the sponge method:

Soak a sponge or some soft cloth in a mixture of 1 cup of water and 1 tablespoon of vinegar (or half a teaspoon of lemon juice). The woman pushes the wet sponge high into her body up to an hour before the couple have sexual relations. She leaves the sponge there for at least 6 hours after having sexual relations.

Breast-feeding

Breast-feeding the baby helps to stop the mother's body from producing eggs for 3–4 months after the baby's birth. After that, some family planning method is needed to prevent pregnancy.

163

(2) *Family planning methods for couples who have definitely decided they do not want any more children*

Surgery on the man

A small operation is done to cut the tubes that carry the sperm to the penis. After this operation the sperm cannot leave the man's body. The operation is simple and painless, and takes only a few minutes. It does not prevent the man from having sexual relations, but only prevents him from making his partner pregnant. (However, a couple will need to use some other method of preventing pregnancy for 3 months after the operation.)

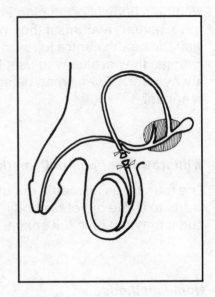

Surgery on the woman

A small simple operation is carried out to remove or tie the tubes that bring the egg to the womb. After the operation the woman will continue to have her monthly period but she cannot become pregnant again. This operation can be done at the local hospital.

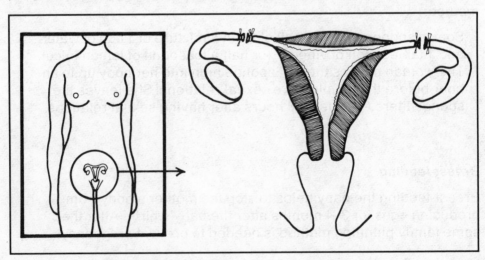

What you can do about common problems

Many women using pills, loops, or injections for the first time may have any of the following:

- a dull backache
- headaches
- a change in the pattern of monthly bleeding
- a feeling of nausea (wanting to vomit).

Explain to these women that:

- their body is getting used to something new
- it may take 6–8 weeks to settle down
- they should take more rest
- if there is no improvement in 6 weeks they should go back to the health centre for a check-up and change the method if necessary.

Send to the health centre any woman who has been using a family planning method and complains of:

- severe bleeding
- swelling and pain in one or both legs
- severe headaches
- no bleeding at all for 3 months.

Also send any woman whose loop has come out. At the health centre she may get another loop or she may choose another method.

Records and follow-up

Whenever possible, and if the community agrees, keep a record of:

- families using a planning method
- types of method being used.

Also, if the community agrees, take supplies of condoms and pills with you when making home visits.

Advice for couples who have no children

Family planning also means helping couples who do not have children and want to have them.

Visit couples who have been living together for 2 years, but have no child, and want to have a child. Encourage them to visit the health centre. Go with them if necessary. Discuss these families with the health service staff, who can give you extra help.

Unit 19

Health problems of women

Women have health problems that men do not have, because women have breasts, a vagina, and a womb.

Few women talk about these parts of their bodies. They discuss health problems of these parts only with other women, when a problem has become serious. They do not often discuss them with their husbands and they do not like to talk about them with other men.

Learning objectives

After studying this unit you should be able to:

1 Explain to women the common health problems that affect them only, and suggest treatment.

2 Find out about the women's health problems in your community.

3 Identify women who need treatment and refer them to the nearest clinic or hospital where women's health problems are treated.

Women's health problems

Lumps in the breast

If a woman who has recently had a baby and has been breast-feeding her baby has a lump in her breast, and one or both of the breasts are sore, see Unit 17.

If a woman feels there are lumps in her breasts at any other time, she must go to the health centre or hospital as soon as possible to see a doctor. Women should feel their breasts regularly and if they find lumps in them they should tell you about them.

The pictures below show how to feel lumps in the breasts. Show these pictures to women so that they can check themselves regularly.

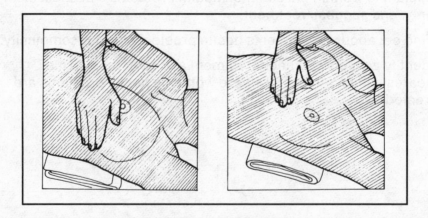

Pain or discomfort during monthly bleeding (*period*)

Healthy women, between the ages of about 13 and 45 years bleed for 4–7 days every month. Every woman's bleeding pattern is slightly different. Some women complain of pain, discomfort, and a feeling of "heaviness" at this time. Suggest the following to relieve pain and discomfort.

- Fill a bottle with hot (not boiling) water and close the cap tightly. Place the bottle over the painful area.

- If the woman does not do hard physical work, ask her to take more exercise.
- Take 2 aspirins to ease the pain.
- Use less salt in food.

If monthly periods do not start

(1) *Before 16 years of age*. Suggest that the young woman be given more to eat, including plenty of green leafy vegetables. Give her iron sulfate tablets (see Annex 1). Find out how much work this young woman does. If she does a lot of work suggest to the family that she should be allowed to do less work.

(2) *After 16 years of age*. Ask the family to take her to the hospital to see a doctor.

Monthly bleeding stops

The woman may be pregnant. Pregnancy is the commonest reason for monthly bleeding to stop in women between 15 and 40 years of age (see Unit 17).

When a woman is more than 45 years old, she gradually stops producing eggs and then she can have no more babies. This is normal.

Monthly bleeding is irregular

(1) In women between 40 and 45 years old the monthly period may sometimes not come, or more than one may come in a month. The woman may also sometimes feel very hot, especially her face, and may sweat a lot. This woman is probably beginning to stop producing eggs. Explain that this is normal. It may go on for 2–3 years, but it will gradually stop.

(2) If a woman of any age bleeds irregularly and she does *not* feel hot, *this may be dangerous*. She may have a lump inside her body which is bleeding. Only a doctor can check this and give her treatment. She may also have swelling and pain in her belly. Send her to the hospital *very soon*.

A woman has heavy bleeding

If a woman has missed one or more monthly periods before the heavy bleeding started, the woman is probably pregnant and the egg that is growing into a baby is trying to come out.

If there is no pain, the pregnancy may be saved by asking the woman to rest in bed immediately. She must not do any work or walk about. If the bleeding stops for one whole day and night, she can get up, but she must continue to rest as much as possible and should do no hard work (such as lifting heavy things) during the rest of her pregnancy. If the bleeding does not stop, take her to the hospital.

If there is pain, it will probably be difficult to save the pregnancy. The pain and bleeding are like a little labour and delivery. Get clean water and soap and ask the woman to wash herself carefully to prevent fever. Place clean cloths on her vulva to catch the blood. Give her plenty to drink, especially rehydration fluid made from salt, sugar and water. Take her to hospital if possible. This is because sometimes only a part of the egg may come out and the woman may bleed a lot. This is very dangerous. Take to the hospital everything that comes out of the woman's body.

If the woman is not pregnant and bleeding heavily, ask her to lie down. Wash her carefully with soap and water. Put clean cloths over her vulva to catch all the blood. Take her to the hospital. Give her many drinks of rehydration fluid (salt, sugar and water) on the journey. Keep her warm.

A woman has pain in her belly

If she is between 14 and 45 years old. Ask her when she had her last monthly period. *Even if she has missed only one period*, she may be pregnant, the egg may be stuck in the egg tube and the tube may have burst. A few spots of blood may come from her genitals. If this has happened, the pain will get worse, she will become very ill, and she may die if she is not taken to hospital. She may need an operation. Explain this to the family.

Make the woman lie down; she must not walk. Keep her warm and give her only sips of water to drink and nothing to eat. Give her half a cup of rehydration fluid (salt, sugar, and water) every half hour. Try to go with her and the family to the hospital and explain to the doctor what has happened.

Discharges and bad smells from the vagina

It is normal for a woman to have a discharge which is clear or slightly yellow.

The discharge is slightly green and smells bad. Ask the woman to:

- wash her genitals carefully with soap and water
- wash her underclothes (boil them if possible and dry them in the hot sun)
- put two teaspoons of lemon juice in a cup of clean water and soak a clean cloth in this, and use it to clean out the inside of the vagina every morning and evening for one week.

The woman can pass this disease to the man, and the man can pass it back to the woman. Therefore, the man must wash his penis with soap and water every day after drawing back the foreskin. If there is no improvement after several days, send both the man and the woman to the health centre for treatment (see also Unit 43).

The discharge is thick white or yellow, and the genitals are very itchy. Treat as above.

The discharge is spotted with blood. The woman should see a doctor as soon as possible.

A woman cannot hold urine or faeces

A difficult childbirth may tear the vagina and the lower end of the gut or the urinary bladder. Faeces or urine may leak out through the vagina. This makes the woman very miserable.

Talk to all women who had long labours and difficult births, to find out if any of them have this problem. Explain to the families that

171

this can be treated in the hospital. Try to persuade all women with this condition to see a doctor soon. After treatment, these women should have their babies in the hospital, and never at home.

Lumps in the belly or vagina

A lump in the belly. If you find a lump in the belly when you examine a non-pregnant woman, or if she tells you she has a lump there, explain to her that:

■ it can be taken out at the hospital

■ it will get bigger if it is not removed

■ she should see the doctor at the hospital soon.

A lump in the vagina. A lump coming out of the vagina, especially when the woman coughs, laughs, or lifts heavy things, usually happens after she has had several babies. She should see a doctor at the hospital, who will probably suggest an operation and exercises.

Finding out about women's problems

When the health worker in the community is a woman, she will find it easy to find out about women's health problems because the women will tell her about them without any difficulty.

When the community health worker is a man he can find out about women's health problems in several ways, for example:

■ by talking to older women in the community who assist at births, and asking their help

■ by discussing these problems with leaders of women's groups, who can then talk to other women

■ by talking to educated women in the community who can pass on the health worker's knowledge to other women

■ by suggesting to men in the community that they come and talk to you about the health problems of their wives and daughters

■ by finding one woman in the community whom all the women respect and using her as an "adviser" and by teaching *her* how to help women.

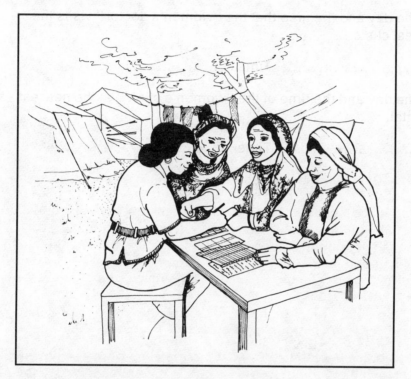

Many women's health problems, particularly those related to irregular monthly bleeding or no monthly bleeding (see page 169), can be prevented by:

■ early care during pregnancy

■ selecting the safest place to deliver the baby

■ spacing pregnancies with intervals of 2 years or more between births, in order to give the mother's body time to become strong again between a birth and the start of the next pregnancy.

Telling women when and where to go to see the women's doctor

Write down in these spaces:

(1) The day and the time that the "women's doctor" visits the nearest clinic.

Day .... Time ....

(2) The day and the time of the "women's clinic" at the nearest hospital.

Day .... Time ....

Chapter 5
Health care of children

Unit 20
Child care and feeding

To grow strong and healthy, children need a lot of healthy food, care, and attention. The weight of a growing child increases a little every month. When the child is not growing properly or is sick, his weight will not increase; it may even decrease. Therefore, if you record the weight of a child every month you can tell whether he is growing properly or not.

When children do not get enough food of the right kind they become sick and stop growing. The mothers must know which foods are good for their children, and how to give those foods to them in a way that they will like.

Remember, breast-feeding is best; bottle-feeding may be dangerous.

Learning objectives

After studying this unit you should be able to:

1 Explain to parents why children should have regular health examinations during the first few years of life.

2 Use the growth chart to discuss with parents a child's growth and what they can do to make sure that the child grows normally.

3 Check the normal development of a child using the major milestones.

4 Identify an underfed child without using a growth chart.

5 Advise mothers about foods that help children to grow and develop normally.

Why children should have regular health examinations

Discuss with parents and women's groups the following points:

(1) If children are to grow up to be strong and healthy their parents and families must care for them and give them attention. By taking them for regular examinations at a health centre the parents can know how well their children are growing.

(2) Proper feeding of children is essential. A baby must eat enough food to make him grow. He cannot grow normally without the right food.

(3) One way to check whether the child is eating enough is by watching his weight. If it goes *up* the family is feeding him well. If the weight does *not* go up, then the family must give the child more of the right kind of food if they want him to grow strong.

(4) A newborn baby can do nothing for itself. As the child's body gets bigger and stronger, he gradually sits up, stands up, begins to walk, begins to talk, etc. Babies who are well fed can do these things when they reach certain ages. Babies who are not well fed, or who are often sick, will grow slowly and will take much longer to learn to do these things.

(5) The family is responsible for the care of its children. Make sure that the whole family knows about the child's needs, which include regular sleep, proper feeding, and time to play. The family should also know about the danger signals of ill health (for example, the child stops growing or has diarrhoea or fever), and should let you know immediately. Your job is to help them to know what to do and how to do it; you cannot do it for them.

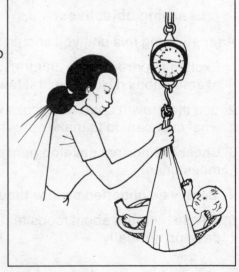

(6) How can you make sure a baby is growing well? The growth chart is a good way of doing this (see

below). To use a growth chart properly, you should know the weight of the baby when it was born. The baby should therefore be weighed on the day he is born or as soon as possible afterwards. You must make sure that each new baby in your village is weighed and that the weight is written on to his growth chart as soon as possible after birth.

Using a growth chart to monitor the weight of children

A growth chart is a record of a child's weight at different ages. To use it properly you must know how to weigh a child correctly on a balance or scale. Set the scale to zero before weighing the child. Each time you weigh a child, make sure he or she is wearing the same sort of clothes (of roughly the same weight). It is best to weigh a child without any clothes, if the weather is not too cold and if the local customs permit this.

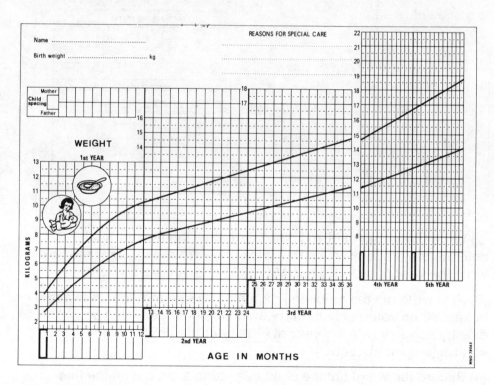

Recording weights on a growth chart

The weight of a child should be recorded on a growth chart according to the instructions given below.

(1) Write the name, address, and other information about the child and the family on the back of the chart. It is important to do this at once to show whose record it is and to avoid recording one child's weight on another child's chart.

APPOINTMENTS

GROWTH CHART

| Health centre | | Child's No. |

Child's name

| Date first seen | Birthday |

| Mother's name | Registration No. |

| Father's name | Registration No. |

Where the family lives (address)

BROTHERS AND SISTERS

Year/birth	Boy/Girl	Remarks	Year/birth	Boy/Girl	Remarks

IMMUNIZATIONS

TUBERCULOSIS Vaccine (BCG) - Date :

DIPHTHERIA, WHOOPING COUGH, TETANUS Vaccine (DPT)

Date : 1ª dose   2ª dose

3ª dose

POLIOMYELITIS Vaccine (OPV)

Date : 1ª dose   2ª dose

3ª dose

MEASLES Vaccine-Date :

OTHER Vaccines (specify with date) :

Has the mother had her tetanus vaccine ?

Date : 1st dose   2nd dose

Repeat dose

(2) Write the month of birth in the box below the first vertical column (the first box which has thick lines around it). Near the box write the year of birth. This is May 1982 in Example 1.

(3) Now write out the following months of the year in the following boxes. When you reach January, write the year near that box exactly as you wrote the year of birth near the box for the month of birth (see instruction 2).

(4) Record the weight of the child by putting a big dot on the line corresponding to that weight. For example, if the weight of a child

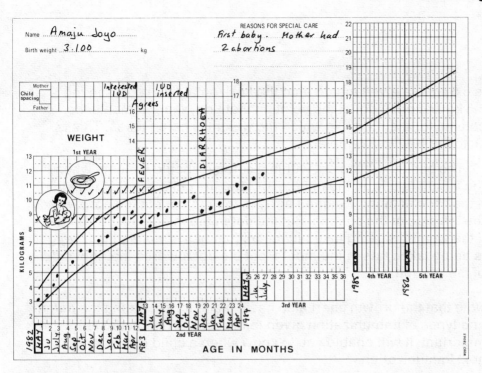

Example 1. Growth chart of a healthy baby

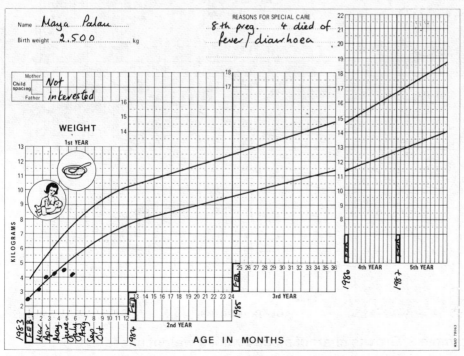

Example 2. Growth chart of a weak baby who has stopped growing

is 6.5 kg in a given month, find the horizontal line representing 6.5 kg and put a dot at the point on that line where it meets the column for the month in which the weight is being taken. This is October 1982 in Example 1.

(5) The position of the dot within a column should indicate when in the month (early, in the middle, or late) the child is being weighed. If the child is being weighed early in the month, put the dot towards the left side of the column. Put the dot in the middle of the column if the weight is being taken in the middle of the month. If the weight is being taken late in the month, put the dot towards the right side of the column.

Note that the growth chart also has a place for recording the dates and types of immunization given to the child. This record is important. It will enable you to know when a child is due for his next immunization.

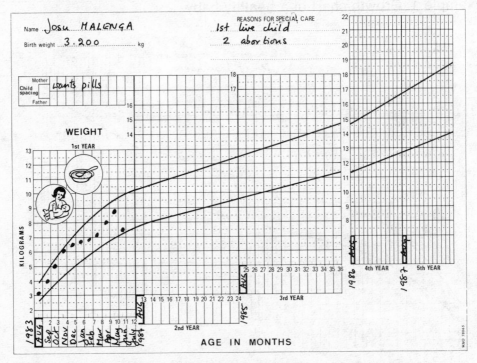

Example 3. Growth chart of a baby whose weight has fallen

The child's weight should be recorded every month for the first 2 years of life. After that, the weight could be recorded every 3 months for up to 5 years of life. The recording of weight up to 5 years is particularly important for children who need special attention (see section on "Identifying underfed children" on page 183).

In judging the growth of a child from a growth chart, remember that the child is growing properly if his weight continues to increase every month. If the growth chart shows that a child's weight has not increased for 2 months or is lower than the previous month's weight, find out the reason for it. The child may have been ill during that month or he may not be getting enough to eat. This child needs care and should go to the health centre for a check up. In the meantime, ask the mother to give the child more food and discuss the problem with the family.

Look at Examples 1, 2, and 3 on the previous pages. Example 1 is the chart of a healthy baby who is growing and developing well. The mother has followed the advice given to her about feeding the child. Examples 2 and 3 are the charts of children who are beginning to lose weight. When you see charts like this you must ask two questions:

(1) *Has the baby been ill recently?* For example, he may have had diarrhoea or fever. When babies are sick they may not want to eat. But parents should know that the child must eat even during sickness (Unit 23). Treat the child if necessary or send him to the health centre.

(2) *What did the child eat yesterday and how many times did he eat?* Find out what and how much the child has been eating. It is possible that the child is not getting the right amount of food for his age. Show the mother the chart, and explain to her that the fall in weight means that:

- the child has stopped growing
- the child needs more food.

Explain to the mother what and how much the child needs to eat to grow normally (see the section on "Feeding children correctly for health, growth, and development" on page 186).

The growth chart also has space for recording any illnesses the child gets (see Example 1). The weight of the child in the month in which he gets the illness will often be lower than the weight in the previous month. If you give the child any treatment for his illness, you should note it on the chart so that when you see him next time you can remember what advice you gave to the family and see how well it worked.

When you find that a child is not growing properly, visit the family and talk to all the adults. The baby belongs not only to the mother, but also to the father. Both parents and other members of the household should know about good child-feeding practices. All can help, and the mother may need your support to make sure that the whole family takes an active interest in the child's development.

The child should be weighed again the next month. If there has been no gain in weight, the parents should take him to the health centre.

Milestones of development

Growth and development

Growth means getting bigger. Development means being able to do more and more things. A child can learn to do more things only when his body is big and strong enough and when his mind is working normally.

There are *four* different milestones in a child's development:

(1) Between 6 and 8 months of age a child can sit without support.

(2) By 18 months a child can walk without support.

(3) By 2 years, a child can say single words in common use, and can show that he knows what they mean. For example, he should be able to say the words for "mother", "grandmother", "dog".

(4) Between $2\frac{1}{2}$ and 3 years of age, a child can say 3 or 4 words together in a short sentence, e.g., "all go market", "daddy gone bus".

Some children cannot do these things at the usual ages. There can
be two reasons for this:

(1) Usually, children who have not been fed correctly cannot do
these things at the ages stated above. Such children will improve
if they are given the right food in the right amount for their age.

(2) A few children cannot do these things even when they have
enough to eat. They are called "slow" children. They are slow to
sit, slow to walk, and slow to talk. When they go to school they
will also be slow to learn. You should refer such children to your
supervisor for advice.

These children may have been born like this, or may have become
like this because of an illness. Sometimes it may be that the family
is not talking or playing with them enough. There are also many
other reasons why children may be slow.

Remember *it is not their fault* that they are slow. Even though they
are slow, they are doing as well as they can. Try to help their
families, friends and teachers to understand this and tell them to
be patient. Such children need to be taught to do things in very
small steps, e.g., at first teach them just to put on one piece of
clothing rather than to dress completely. (Even this may take
several weeks.) Teaching such children takes longer, but very often
they can learn. These children need to be praised for trying to do
the right thing even if they do not succeed.

Identifying underfed children

Underfed children must be examined and weighed regularly. Some
families may be living so far away from your house that you may
not be able to see their babies regularly. If some babies of the
families that live far from you are underweight, you must make a
special effort to see them.

You may also be able to see some of the children you do not see
regularly at the village market when families come to buy things
or at village festivals.

Children who need special attention are described on pages 184–186.

Children who are all skin and bones and look like old persons

These children have not been getting enough food. They are often ill. Their bodies are very weak and they get tired very easily. They are so weak that they do not want to eat; eating is hard work for them. They are very ill and need special help at a feeding centre or hospital till they are strong enough to eat properly. The mothers of such children will need help in preparing special foods for them.

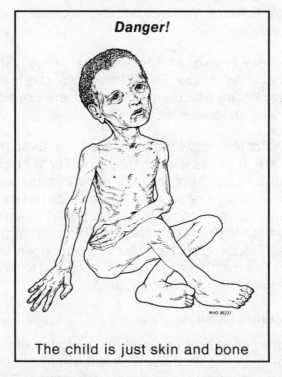

Danger!

WHO 86231

The child is just skin and bone

Children who are swollen, have swollen bellies, arms and legs, look miserable and have no energy

Such children are eating too little or eating the wrong kinds of food. Their bodies swell with water instead of muscle. They should be referred immediately to the feeding centre or health centre or hospital.

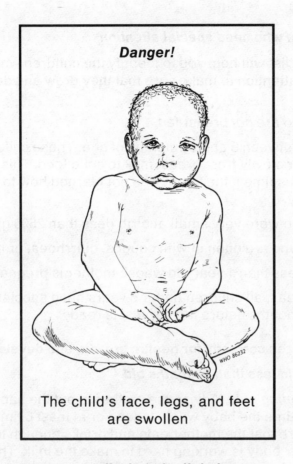

Danger!

The child's face, legs, and feet
are swollen

WHO 86232

Children who cannot see well when the light is poor

These children stumble and cannot walk about in the dark. This is
called "night blindness". This condition should be treated quickly
otherwise the child may become blind. A child with night blindness
needs vitamin A immediately: give retinol (see Annex 1). If you
have no retinol, the child should be taken to the health centre as
soon as possible. To prevent night blindness all children should eat
fruit and vegetables that are yellow, orange, or red (such as
oranges, carrots, etc.). See also Unit 37.

Other children who need special attention

The following list will help you to identify the children who need your special attention to make sure that they grow and develop properly:

(1) Babies who are *not* breast-fed.

(2) Children between 6 and 24 months of age. These children are changing over slowly from breast milk to solid food. This can be a very dangerous time if the family has not learned how to feed the child correctly.

(3) Babies who were very small at birth (less than 2500 g).

(4) Children who are often ill with coughs, diarrhoea, or malaria.

(5) Children less than 1 year old whose mother is pregnant again.

(6) In rural areas, all children under 5 years need special care during the 2 months before the harvest is ready.

Feeding children correctly for health, growth, and development

Feeding a child less than 5 months old

(1) *Breast-feeding only*. Advise the mother to put the baby to the breast every time the baby wants to feed or at least 6 times every day. Make sure that the mother eats and drinks enough to make good milk. Her body is working hard to make the milk. Therefore, she should do less work in the fields and at home.

(2) *Bottle-feeding.*

- Bottle-fed babies are more likely to get sick than breast-fed babies. This is because it is difficult for mothers to boil bottles and teats to keep them clean. Also, mothers may not know how to make the feeds correctly. A baby needs 5–6 feeds a day and many mothers do not have time to boil the bottles, teats, and water every time they make a feed. If bottles, teats and water are not boiled there is a very high risk of the baby becoming ill.

- Bottle-fed babies are likely to be underfed because many parents may not know how much powdered milk should be put in one feed. Parents often forget that a growing baby needs more and

186

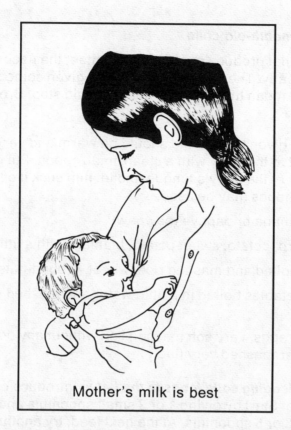

Mother's milk is best

more milk. Also, very often parents do not put enough powdered milk in the feeds because the milk is very expensive. This means that the baby does not get enough food to grow properly.

■ All bottle-fed babies must be taken to a health centre once every month. There, they can be treated for illnesses and the mother can be told to increase gradually the amount of milk and water as the baby grows. At the health centre the parents will also be told about what other foods are good for the baby.

Remember!

In the first 4 months of life, breast-milk is the best food for babies.

Feeding a 5-month-old child

A mother cannot produce enough milk to meet the needs of a 5-month-old baby. The baby should now be given some solid foods. This does *not* mean that breast-feeding should stop. Breast-feeding *must* continue.

The first food given to the child should be warm and very soft. It should be fed to the baby with a clean small spoon. Put the spoon of food on *top* of the baby's tongue and let him suck it off. Any of the following foods may be used:

- mashed banana or papaya (pawpaw)
- mashed taro, potato, sweet potato, plantain with a little oil
- very well boiled and mashed rice, wheat, ground-nuts, lentils
- green vegetables boiled in a little water and mashed *with* the water
- soft-boiled eggs, very soft mashed fish without any bones, or well cooked liver mashed very finely.

How to start feeding solid foods to the baby. Introduce only one new food at a time. Start by giving 1 or 2 small spoonfuls and increase gradually to 5 or 6 spoonfuls. At the next feed, try another sort of food. Always give the solid food *before* breast-feeding, when the baby is hungry.

A baby will not eat spicy food at first. He may be between 1 and 2 years old before he can do so. Warn mothers that when a baby spits out new food, it is *not* because he does not like it but because it has a new taste.

Give the solid food before the breast-feed at the same time every day for a week. The next week give some solid food before a second breast-feed. Repeat this during the third and the fourth weeks.

At 6 months the baby should have 4–5 teaspoons of mashed food before a breast-feed, 4 times every day, and at least 2 breast-feeds without solid food.

Feeding babies older than 6 months of age

The mother will have seen by now that the baby can eat most of the food she offers him. Remind her that the baby can grow bigger only if he gets enough to eat. A six-month-old baby needs solid food *and* breast milk 4 times a day *plus* breast milk without extra food 2 or more times a day.

At least twice a day the baby's food should contain:

- One or more of the foods that babies need in order to grow normally. These are meat, fish, eggs, beans, lentils.

- One or more of the energy-giving foods. These are potato, rice, plantain, taro, cassava.

- Foods that prevent night blindness and protect the child against infections. These are fruit and vegetables.

See also the section on foods for pregnant women in Unit 15.

Feeding a child who is more than 1 year old

By one year, the child is gradually beginning to eat like an adult, and the mother's milk is no longer sufficient. Advise the mother to take great care that the child eats well, and to add gradually to the diet such foods as butter, ground-nut oil, palm oil, cotton oil, wheat oil, coconut oil. The baby should eventually eat all types of food that the family eats.

Remind all mothers to have the children weighed regularly

When growth charts are kept up to date, mothers can see how well their children are growing and how well they are feeding them. You should see more often the children who need special attention (see page 184) and those whose growth curve is not following the correct path.

Children who are completely normal will not need your special attention and can be weighed less often.

Unit 21

Protecting against infectious diseases: immunization [1]

Infectious diseases cause many deaths in children. These diseases are caused by germs that attack the body and that can be passed from person to person.

The body can protect itself against some germs when the person is "immunized". Immunization means that a drug called a "vaccine" is injected into the body or swallowed (the poliomyelitis vaccine is swallowed) to protect against possible attacks by germs.

Six common infectious diseases can be prevented by immunization: tuberculosis, diphtheria, whooping cough, tetanus, poliomyelitis, and measles.

Check with your supervisor the local names of these diseases. Always use these local names when talking to the people about the diseases. See also the glossary on page 415.

Learning objectives

After studying this unit you should be able to:

1 Find out which children and pregnant women need to be immunized against the common infectious diseases.

2 Inform the community why, how, when, and where children and pregnant women should be immunized.

3 Assist in the preparation of immunization sessions.

4 Keep simple records for immunization purposes.

---

[1] Immunization and vaccination mean the same thing.

190

Who needs to be immunized against the six common diseases?

- All children under 1 year of age.
- Other children who have not been fully immunized.

Also, immunization against tetanus should be given to:

- every pregnant woman to protect her baby from getting this disease after birth, and
- all other women who are of child-bearing age and have not been immunized previously against tetanus.

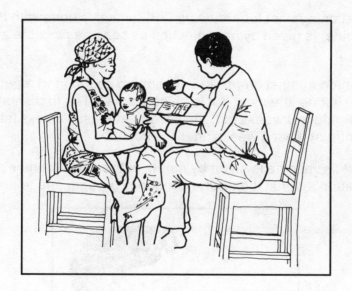

What do people need to know about vaccines and infectious diseases?

Why get immunized?

The community needs to know that young children and those women who are going to have children soon can be protected from 6 infectious diseases (always use their local names). These diseases are very dangerous and can cause death, *but they can be prevented by immunization.*

Parents should not be afraid to have their children immunized. The injections cause only very little pain for a moment, but these dangerous diseases can handicap children for their whole lives, or even kill them.

How and when to get immunized?

A baby cannot be fully immunized against all the 6 diseases in only one visit: the mother must take her child to the health centre at least three times. You should make all mothers understand this so that they will bring back their children when they are requested to do so.

Immunization against *tuberculosis* (TB) (which is done with the BCG vaccine) is given by one injection as soon as possible after birth.

Immunization against *diphtheria*, *whooping cough*, and *tetanus* is combined in one injection, but is given 3 times. The first should be when the child is 6 weeks old, the second at least 4 weeks later, and the third at least 4 weeks after the second.

Poliomyelitis vaccine is given by mouth at the same 3 times as the immunization against diphtheria, whooping cough, and tetanus.

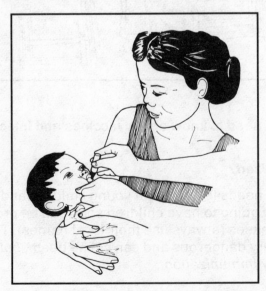

Immunization against *measles* is given by one injection when the child is 9 months old.

A pregnant woman should be immunized by 2 injections of the tetanus vaccine. The first is given as soon as the pregnancy is known, and the second 4 weeks later. (Only one injection is needed when the woman has been vaccinated previously.)

Where can children and women be immunized?

Immunization sessions are organized in your area according to instructions from the national or district health services.

There are two possibilities (ask your supervisors):

■ women take their children to the health centre, or

■ a health team comes periodically to the village to immunize those who are due to be immunized.

Important!

It may happen that mothers are sent back from the health centre because there is no vaccine or that the health workers do not come on the promised day and time. If that is the case, then the health care for women and children in your community is bad. You have a duty to complain to your supervisor. If that does not help, you should complain to the village or district authorities. Tell them that the women and the children in your community are not getting the proper care to which they are entitled.

How can you assist in preparing for immunization sessions?

When women have to take their children to a health centre, you can assist by:

■ finding out the place, the day, and the time of the immunization session

■ informing all mothers when to go and where to go, and making sure that they go

■ checking regularly the growth charts of children to make sure that they and the mothers have received the immunizations they need.

When a special immunization team comes to your community, you can assist by:

■ finding out the date and time when the team is supposed to come

■ discussing with the community leaders:

— where to organize the sessions (in a sheltered place, with water, soap, light, etc.)
— what equipment will be needed (tables, chairs, benches)
— how, when, and where to inform and bring together the mothers and children who need immunization

■ reviewing and preparing your records (see below)

■ preparing the waiting area, to make mothers and children as comfortable as possible

■ organizing the queue at the entrance

■ following the instructions of the team and making yourself available.

What records should a community health worker keep for immunizations?

Whenever possible, you should keep three lists:

(1) A list of children born in the community, with their names, dates

of birth, and addresses and the immunizations they have already received.

(2) A list of all pregnant women with their names, addresses, expected dates of delivery, dates of previous immunizations.

(3) A list of all children over 1 year of age who have not been completely immunized.

These lists should be updated every month (see also Unit 51).

Unit 22

Preventing accidents involving children

Accidents are common among children and young people. Some are serious and may kill. Many accidents leave permanent scars or make people handicapped for life. You and the community should try to prevent these serious accidents.

Learning objectives

After studying this unit you should be able to:

1 Explain to families the main causes of accidents at the different stages of childhood and adolescence.

2 Tell them what the community can do to prevent accidents involving children.

3 Suggest what you can do to prevent common accidents in childhood.

The main accidents in childhood

In small children, who crawl and toddle unsafely in and around the house, the common accidents are:

- cuts, burns from fire, and scalds from boiling water or boiling oil

- falls, with wounds or fractures, from climbing or when running

- poisoning from drinking kerosene, petrol, chemicals, etc. or from eating insecticides, rat poison, poisonous berries, pills or tablets, etc.

- drowning in rivers, lakes, ponds, or wells.

In older children, who go around the whole neighbourhood, the common accidents are:

- The same as for young children, but often more serious because older children take more risks. They climb higher in trees or on walls, run faster, and go further into rivers, lakes or the sea.

- Road traffic accidents (which are becoming a main cause of serious accidents) caused by falling from bicycles or being hit by cars on the road.

Among teenagers, who are generally daring and do dangerous things to show off, the most common accidents are traffic accidents. These are the main cause of serious injuries and death among young people. Accidents happen when teenagers drive motorcycles or cars very fast, or when young people are hit by motor vehicles.

The community can do many things to prevent accidents among children

The government can set speed limits for road traffic or set minimum and maximum ages for driving.

The community can:

- fill in old, empty wells

- put fences or barriers around dangerous places

- warn the people by signs

197

- provide services to rescue and care for persons who have accidents
- arrange for children to be taught about accidents at school.

Families can look after their children properly, particularly to prevent home accidents, and can teach them how to avoid accidents.

To understand how accidents can be prevented, let us take an example of a young child alone by a pond who does not know how to swim. Think of what can be done to prevent drowning:

(1) *Get rid of the risk*, for example, by filling in the pond if it is small enough.

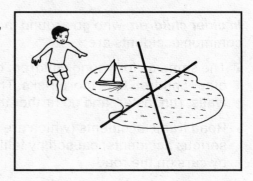

(2) *Cut off the risk*, for example, by putting a fence around it so that the child cannot go near it.

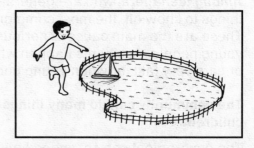

(3) *Keep the child away* from the pond and *watch* him carefully.

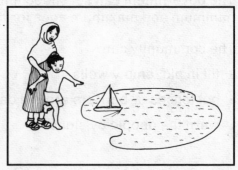

(4) *Inform and remind* the child of the possible dangers by placing warnings — signs, posters at the pond and by oral messages.

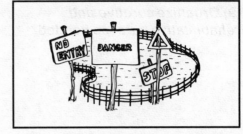

(5) *Teach the child* how to swim.

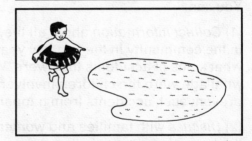

(6) *Give the child safety equipment*, such as floats, a rubber ring, a cork belt, or an inflated tube.

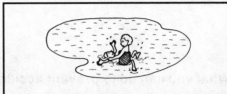

(7) *Provide life-belts at places of high risk.* These may be bathing places, beaches, bridges, ponds, etc.

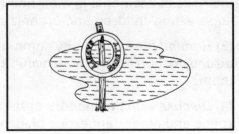

(8) *Provide special supervision and rescue services.*

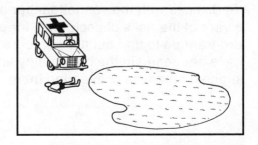

(9) *Organize curative and rehabilitative care*, as needed.

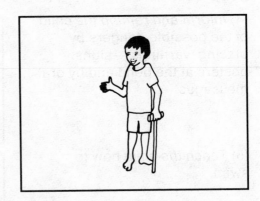

What you can do to prevent accidents among children

You can:

(1) *Collect information* about all the accidents that have happened in the community in the last few years. Find out how many and what kinds of accidents they were. Where did they happen and what age were the children involved? Has anything been done to prevent such accidents from happening again?

(2) *Discuss* with families and women's groups how they can reduce the risks of accidents in their homes and in other places by supervising children and organizing play areas.

(3) *Remind* the community committee about the accidents that have already occurred and may occur again if nothing is done to prevent them.

(4) *Discuss* with the leaders or the committee how to make the roads and other dangerous places safe for the people.

(5) *Discuss* with the schoolteacher how to make children more aware of the risks of accidents, for example, by organizing a programme to find out the numbers and types of accidents that have happened in the community and by asking the children to suggest means of preventing them.

Unit 23
Care of a sick child

Most children get sick sometimes.

Well fed children get sick less often than badly fed children. Badly fed children become sick more seriously than well fed children.

Children who work too many hours a day and do not get enough time to play or sleep may get sick more often.

Full immunization prevents most of the diseases that kill very young children.

Early treatment can stop a sickness from becoming dangerous. A sick child needs to eat and drink to help the body to fight the sickness.

A sick child needs more care than a sick adult. Never leave a sick child alone.

Learning objectives

After studying this unit you should be able to:

1 Explain to the families what are the common serious sicknesses of children.

2 Help a mother to look after a sick child at home.

3 Decide which sick children should be sent to the health centre or hospital.

A child who refuses to eat or drink and who does not want to play may be at the beginning of a sickness: watch the child carefully.

When a sick child does not get good care early, the sickness may become dangerous. It is important to treat children early.

Children who are weak and of low weight become sick more easily.

Your community may have very strong ideas about how to care for sick children. Find out what they are. Some may be dangerous and may make the child more sick. Always make sure that a sick child:

■ eats and drinks enough (except when there is belly pain)

■ is kept warm

■ is washed every day.

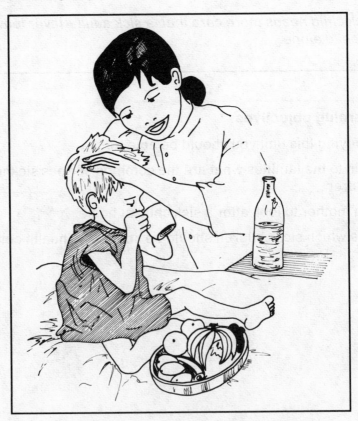

Common serious sicknesses in children

Tetanus of the newborn

If a dirty or rusted blade or scissors is used to cut the cord, the baby may get tetanus. The germs enter the baby's body through the cord. First, the baby's arms and legs become stiff. Then he has difficulty in opening his mouth, and soon he cannot open it at all. A baby with tetanus can be treated only in a hospital. In most cases the babies die, but this disease can be prevented by:

- immunizing the pregnant mother (see Units 15 and 21)
- making sure that all birth attendants cut the cord with a clean, new blade, dress it *only* with very clean material and do not put any powder or other material on the cord or navel.

Infectious diseases

Tetanus, diphtheria, whooping cough, polio, measles and tuberculosis can be prevented by immunization (see Unit 21). Without full immunization children may get these sicknesses, they may become very sick, and may even die. They may also pass them to other children.

Diarrhoea

Diarrhoea is a very serious disease in small children (see also Unit 26). Breast-fed babies rarely get diarrhoea. Diarrhoea happens when dirt or dirty water or food get inside the child's body.

To prevent and treat diarrhoea, ask mothers to

- continue breast-feeding
- give solid food at least 4 times a day—the food should be made easy to eat by mashing it or making it into soup
- give one glass of rehydration fluid (mixture of salt, sugar, and water) every time the child passes a watery stool
- take the child to the health centre if the diarrhoea is not better in 2 days; take plenty of rehydration fluid for the journey.

Care at home

A child with fever

When a person has fever it means that his body is fighting an infection. Children may have very high fever (see also Unit 24).

When a child has a fever:

- Keep the body cool by sponging it often with cool water.

- Put only one cotton shirt on the child and cover the child in the cot or bed with a cotton cover. Too many clothes will make the child too warm.

- A child with fever should drink as much as possible. Rehydration fluid is good, but the child can also have tea or fruit juice or milk.

- Give aspirin according to the child's age (see Annex 1).

- An adult should always look after a sick child. A sick child should not be left alone.

- As soon as the fever goes down, give the child plenty to eat. Fighting a sickness makes the body tired and only good food can make the child strong again.

- If the fever does *not* go down after 1 full day and 1 full night, the parents should take the child to the health centre for more treatment.

A child who coughs

Coughing is the body's way of trying to clear blockages in the lungs or air-tubes or throat (see also Unit 25). Many coughs can be prevented by keeping a child's nose clean. The stuff that runs out of his nose by day may run into his lungs when he sleeps. Teach all children to blow their nose to keep it clean.

Encourage children to run and jump. This is good exercise for their lungs and will keep them healthy.

When a child has a cough:

- sit him up in bed or against a wall, with pillows.

- cover the chest with loose light clothes only. Heavy or tight clothes will make it hard for the lungs to work and the cough will get worse.

- give small meals, 4–5 times a day, to help the body fight the cough.

- give plenty of drinks.

Take a coughing child to the health centre if:

- the cough does not improve in 3–4 days

- there is loss of weight

- there is high fever

- anyone in the house or family has tuberculosis (TB).

A sick child uses a lot of energy to fight the sickness. After the sickness the child needs to make his body strong again. To do this he will need:

- to eat good food 3–4 times every day

- to eat plenty of fruit and vegetables

- to do less work than usual for 2–3 weeks.

The child should have a check up at the health centre to make sure that he is gaining weight again.

Chapter 6
Treating sick people

Unit 24
Fever

A person whose temperature is over 37.5 °C has fever. (C is the abbreviation for centigrade or Celsius.)

A child under school age whose temperature is over 38 °C may be very ill.

Fever, like diarrhoea, makes the patient lose a lot of water.

Learning objectives

After studying this unit you should be able to:

1 Tell whether a person has fever.

2 Discuss with people in the community how germs attack and enter the body.

3 Advise people how to protect themselves against germs.

4 Decide what to do with a patient who has fever:

- for less than 24 hours
- for more than 3 days
- with other signs.

How do people get fever

A person gets fever when his body is attacked by very small living things called germs.

Germs live in the air, soil, water, and infected animals or people. They can enter the body through:

- the air we breathe
- unclean food and drink
- the skin (from wounds, bites of mosquitos and other insects or of dogs)
- sexual contact with infected people.

How can people protect themselves against germs

To protect against germs, people should:

- eat clean fresh food
- drink only safe or boiled water or other safe or boiled fluids
- wash their hands before eating
- wash their hands after defecating
- avoid contact with people who have acute infectious disease
- avoid sexual contact with people who may have venereal disease
- keep the surroundings of their houses and villages clean
- protect themselves against bites of insects and animals
- be immunized against the common infectious diseases.

What should you do when a patient has fever?

When you think a patient may have fever, take his temperature (see Annex 2, page 385). If it is above 37.5 °C, ask for how long the patient has had fever.

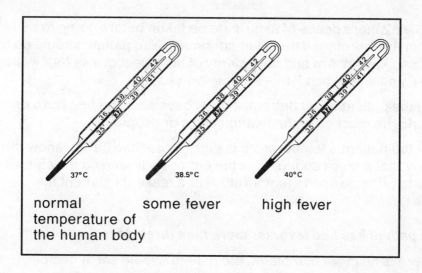

normal
temperature of
the human body

some fever

high fever

The patient has had fever for less than 24 hours and he has no other complaint

(1) Ask if he has been in an area where there is malaria. If yes, start treatment at once (see Annex 1). (Chloroquine is the usual treatment for malaria, but in many places, chloroquine may not be suitable. You must learn from your supervisor or the health centre how to treat and prevent malaria in your country or district.)

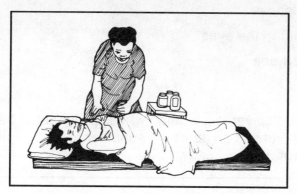

(2) If there is no malaria in your area, give 2 aspirins if the patient is an adult, and less if the patient is a small child (see dosages in Annex 1); ask the patient to take the aspirin at once.

(3) Give 2 more doses of aspirin (to be taken before going to bed and in the morning) if the fever continues. The patient should go to bed and keep warm and take plenty of hot sweet drinks (tea, water, milk), and a little salt if there is much sweating.

(4) If the patient is not better within $1\frac{1}{2}$ days after the first dose of aspirin, he must go to the health centre or hospital.

(5) If the patient's temperature is high (more than 39 °C), show the family that a quick sponging of the entire body with cool water will help to bring down the temperature and make the patient feel better.

The patient has had fever for more than three days

If there is no other complaint, the patient should see a doctor or go to hospital without more delay.

The patient has fever and another complaint

Send the patient to hospital at once if as well as fever he has any of the following complaints:

- stiff neck
- severe pain
- unconsciousness
- yellow colour in the eyes
- severe diarrhoea
- convulsions.

If the patient with fever is a woman who is pregnant or has recently had a baby or has had an abortion, send her to the hospital at once (see also Chapter 4).

Remember!

A patient with fever should drink plenty of water, because he will lose a lot of water by sweating.

Unit 25
Cough

Usually when someone starts to cough, it means that he or she has an infection in the nose and throat. In most cases the infection is mild and the patient gets better after some days without treatment. Sometimes in small children the infection may become more severe and you will need to treat such children. In yet other cases the infection may even spread to the lungs. This can be very dangerous, especially if the child is underfed and weak.

You should know when a child with a cough has a mild, moderate, or severe infection, and what to do in each case. Also, you should help the people to take action to prevent diseases that cause coughing.

Learning objectives

After studying this unit you should be able to:

1 Tell whether a child (or another person) with a cough has a mild, moderate, or severe infection.

2 Show the family how to care for a child who is coughing.

3 Treat a child with a severe cough.

4 Talk to the community about what can be done to prevent coughing diseases.

Care of a child or an older person who is coughing

A mild infection

The cough may sound bad, but if the child feels well, does not want to lie down, and is eating and drinking normally he probably has only a mild infection. He may have a running nose or his nose may be blocked, and he may have a hoarse voice.

Explain to the family that the child should take plenty of fluids and as much food as he wants. If this is a baby who is breast-feeding, the mother should continue to breast-feed. A baby whose nose is blocked will not be able to breathe or suck easily. Show the mother how to clear the nose: use a damp piece of cotton and twist it into each nostril to get the thick discharge out. Then, with the child's head back, put 2–3 drops of salty water into each nostril.

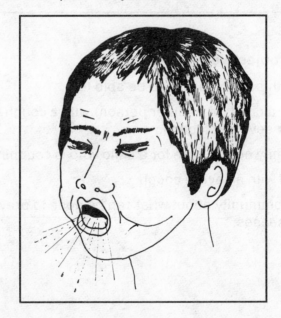

If there is fever, give aspirin for 3 days (see dosage in Annex 1).

A moderate infection

If the child has a thick, yellowish discharge from the nose, or he coughs up such a discharge from the throat, he has a moderate infection. Show the mother how to clean the child's nose, with a piece of cotton wool or paper, or a leaf, which should then be burned. The nose should be cleaned whenever it is blocked, and especially before the child goes to sleep and on waking up.

The child may also have a sore throat and earache (pain in the ear), and there may be a discharge of pus from the ear. He may not want to eat and may have no energy. There may be a rash which may spread over the whole body. They may also be some fever (less than 40 °C).

Treat the child with procaine benzylpenicillin (see dosage in Annex 1). If you have no penicillin, treat with sulfamethoxazole + trimethoprim (for dosage see Annex 1). If the child has fever, give aspirin (for dosage, see Annex 1).

The child should rest sitting up in bed and, if possible, away from other children. A baby feeding on breast milk should continue to be breast-fed. The mother should clean the baby's nose before each feed. An older child should have as much to drink as possible, and should continue to take food.

If there is a discharge from the ear, wipe it off the skin with a damp cloth. When the child is better he should be taken to the health centre to have the ear examined by a doctor. The child should sleep with the bad ear on the pillow. This will help the discharge to drain out.

A severe infection

In a severe infection, the child has the same signs as above but he is more sick. The cough will be more severe, and you will be able to hear the child breathing in and out. The openings of the nose (the nostrils) will widen with each breath, and the lips and nails may look blue. There will be high fever (over 40 °C). A young child may have one or more fits (see Unit 45).

This child is dangerously ill and should be taken to hospital immediately. If possible, give procaine benzylpenicillin by injection (see Annex 1) before leaving for hospital.

Prevention of diseases that cause cough

Immunization

Four diseases that cause coughing are whooping cough, measles, diphtheria, and tuberculosis. These can be prevented by immunization. If the immunization service is working well in your district, and you and the community make sure that all babies are fully immunized, no child is likely to get these diseases (see also Unit 21).

Proper feeding

Breast-feeding prevents coughing diseases in babies or makes the disease less severe.

If you can reduce the number of badly fed children in your community, you will reduce the number of severe coughing diseases. Make sure that everybody in the community knows this; repeat it as often as necessary (see also Unit 20).

Keeping the air clean

The parents and other people in the household should not smoke in places where young children are present. The smoke from the cooking fire in the house can also cause coughing diseases. Discuss with all the families how smoke from cooking can be reduced in the house. The air in the house should be free of smoke from a cooking fire, cigarettes, and tobacco.

Smoking can cause coughing and other dangerous diseases in adults. Advise people not to smoke.

Avoiding contact with people who have coughing diseases

Older children and adults with a coughing disease should keep away from young children. They should cover their mouth with a cloth when they cough or sneeze and always turn their head away from other people.

People who cough up sputum should spit it into something that can be burned, such as a cloth, paper, leaf, or a paper box.

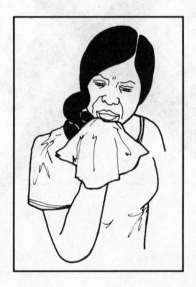

Send to the health centre all patients who have a long-lasting cough

Explain to people who have had a cough for 3 weeks or more that the health centre could examine and treat them, and that this could stop others in the family from getting the cough (see also Unit 11).

Informing parents and the community about coughing diseases

Teach mothers of young children how to know when a coughing disease is serious or dangerous, and what to do in that case. Discuss with the community leaders and groups what could be done to prevent the spread of coughing diseases.

If a lot of people smoke in your community, discuss with community leaders how to prevent young people from taking up this bad habit.

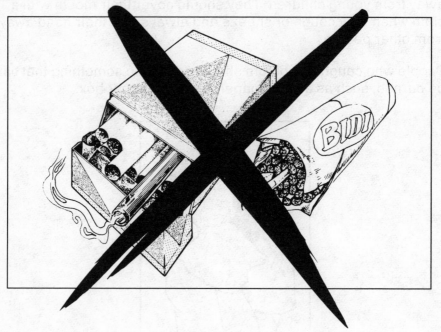

Unit 26

Diarrhoea

When a person passes at least 3 watery stools in a day, he has diarrhoea.

A patient with diarrhoea loses water and salt, may become dehydrated and very weak, and may die if he is not treated.

For treatment, the patient should drink a mixture of water, salt, and sugar. The patient should continue to eat so as not to lose strength.

Diarrhoea is more dangerous in children because they become dehydrated very quickly. All mothers should know about this danger.

Learning objectives

After studying this unit you should be able to:

1 Tell whether a person has diarrhoea.

2 Describe to people the 4 ways in which they may get diarrhoea.

3 Recognize whether or not a person with diarrhoea is dehydrated.

4 Prepare drinks that prevent a person with diarrhoea from becoming dehydrated.

5 Prepare a solution of oral rehydration salts (ORS) when a patient has become dehydrated.

6 Decide what to do when a person has diarrhoea and:
   ■ no other complaint or sign
   ■ other complaints or signs.

7 Advise people on how to prevent diarrhoea.

How people get diarrhoea

Diarrhoea is caused by germs that enter the body through:

- dirty drinking-water—for example, from a dirty pond or river, an unprotected spring or well, or water kept in a dirty container (see Unit 4);

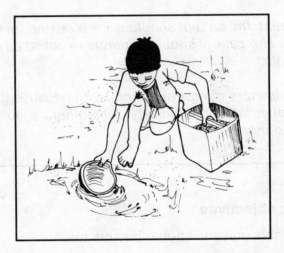

- dirty food—for example, badly washed food, cooked food left outside or in a warm place for too long, or food not protected against dirt, flies, and animals;

- unsafe foods—ones that have not been cooked long enough, such as meat;

- dirty hands—for example, when food is eaten without properly washing hands after defecating or after work.

How to recognize that a person with diarrhoea is dehydrated

With diarrhoea, a patient loses water and salts that the body needs. This quickly weakens the body. This water and these salts should be replaced very quickly. People who have lost too much water and salts are said to be *dehydrated.*

The signs of severe dehydration are:

- the patient is very thirsty

- the eyes appear to be sunken

- the mouth and tongue are dry

- when the skin is pinched, the skinfold remains raised for a few seconds instead of falling back again at once

- the pulse is rapid.

In the case of a child less than 18 months old, the soft spot on the top of the head is sunk in.

Preventing dehydration

It is usually possible to prevent a person with diarrhoea from becoming dehydrated. As soon as diarrhoea starts, people should drink fluids to replace the water and salt they lose. They should drink clean water with salt and sugar as explained below, or any other available household drink which has salt and sugar.

Dehydration in small children

When the patient is a child you should be very careful. A child with diarrhoea becomes dehydrated very quickly and may die in a few hours. The child should *at once* (that is, even before there are signs of dehydration) start to drink the rehydration fluid (mixture of water, salt and sugar) and continue to take a cupful (200 ml)[1] of it for every stool.

How to prepare rehydration fluid

If the mother does not know how to prepare the rehydration fluid, show her or another person caring for the child, how to do it.

If you give enough oral rehydration fluid you will prevent the body from losing all its water (dehydration); in most cases, the diarrhoea will soon stop *without any other treatment.*

---

[1] ml is the abbreviation for millilitre.

Method for making rehydration fluid

Wash your hands with soap and water. Put into a clean bottle:

(1) a three-finger pinch of salt

(2) a four-finger scoop of sugar

(3) 1/2 litre of clean water (boiled if possible).

Shake the bottle well to dissolve the salt and sugar.

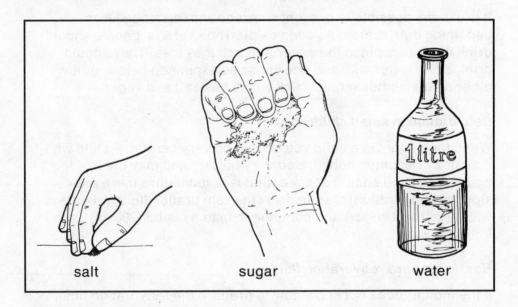

salt   sugar   water

Dehydration in adults

If the patient is an adult, show him how to prepare the rehydration fluid. It should taste less salty than tears.

Teach all mothers of young children how to make a mixture of water, salt and sugar. They should not wait until a child has diarrhoea to learn how to make it. As soon as diarrhoea starts they should begin treatment with this mixture and continue it until the diarrhoea has stopped.

How to treat dehydration

If the patient *has become* dehydrated, treat him by following the instructions given below. (See pages 218-219 for signs of dehydration.)

(1) You should immediately prepare for him a solution with oral rehydration salts (ORS) using one of the ORS packets you have.

Method

- *Wash your hands.*

- *Measure 1 litre [or correct amount for packet used] of clean drinking-water into a clean container. It is best to boil and cool the water, but if this is not possible, use the cleanest water available. Use whatever container you can get, such as a jar, pot, or bottle.*

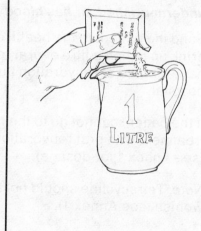

- *Pour all the powder from one packet into the water and mix well until the powder is completely dissolved.*

- *Make your patient drink some of the ORS solution at once. He should continue to drink it as often and as much as he wants (at least 1 litre per 24 hours until the diarrhoea stops).*

Fresh ORS solution should be mixed each day in a clean container. The container should be kept covered. Any solution remaining from the day before should be thrown away.

(2) If you have no ORS packets, prepare a rehydration fluid yourself, following the method described on page 220.

Signs to look for during diarrhoea

The patient has diarrhoea but no other signs

A patient who has diarrhoea but no fever, no blood in the stools, and no other serious complaints should:

- drink the rehydration fluid as indicated above, and
- continue to eat as usual.

The diarrhoea should stop or become very much less within 36 hours; if not, send the patient to the health centre.

The patient has diarrhoea and also a high fever (over 39 °C), or is undernourished, or has blood in the stools.

Send the patient to the health centre or hospital, but first make him drink up to half a litre of oral rehydration fluid. The patient should have a bottle of rehydration fluid to drink during the journey to hospital.

If the patient cannot go to the hospital or health centre, continue treatment with oral rehydration fluid and give tetracycline tablets (see Annex 1 for dosage).

Note: Tetracycline should not be given to children or to pregnant women (see Annex 1).

See the patient again on the third day. If the diarrhoea is better or has stopped, tell the patient to complete the course of treatment with tetracycline and advise him to eat as usual.

Be careful!

If, at any time, there are more patients (particularly adults) than usual with diarrhoea, closely one after the other, or if there are deaths from diarrhoea, there may be an epidemic (see Unit 2). Report at once to the supervisor or health centre.

How to prevent diarrhoea

People can prevent diarrhoea if they learn how it is caused and what action they can take to deal with its causes.

They can stop diarrhoea and can save children from dying from it, if they learn from you how to treat it.

To prevent diarrhoea in your community explain to the people, especially to families with young children, what to do and how to do it. The people should:

KNOW: Water taken from a spring, well, pond, or river that has been polluted by people or animals contains the germs of diarrhoea.

DO: If possible, always boil such water before using it for drinking or cooking.

Discuss with the community leaders or committee how to prevent pollution of the water (see Unit 4).

Work together with the community committee and the leaders and others to make sure that the community has a safe source of water for drinking and cooking.

KNOW: Food carries the germs of diarrhoea when:

- it is not fresh
- it is left in a warm place
- it is exposed to flies, insects, rats and other animals.

DO: Do not cook or eat such food.

Protect all food from contamination (see Unit 5).

KNOW: Food can carry the germs of diarrhoea when it is not properly cooked.

DO: Always cook food well and eat it soon after it has been cooked.

KNOW: Hands carry the germs of diarrhoea when they are not properly washed after defecation or after work.

DO: Always wash hands well (with soap and water, if possible):

- after defecating and after work
- before cooking, serving food, and eating
- before feeding children.

Headaches

People have headaches for many reasons. Most headaches are not serious, but some headaches may be due to a serious disease.

Learning objectives

After studying this unit you should be able to:

1 Ask people questions to decide if a headache is serious or not.

2 Decide what to do in either case.

How to find out whether the headache is serious

Ask the patient:

- How long has he or she had a headache?

- How often does it come?

- How long does it last?

- Has the patient any other complaint or sign of disease?

- If the patient is a woman, is she pregnant?

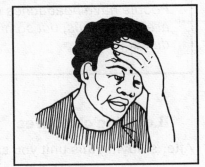

Headaches that are not serious

If the patient does not have a fever or a stiff neck (see below), and is not behaving strangely, the headache is most probably not serious. It may be one of two types of headache described below.

(1) *Some headaches often come and go* for weeks or months. They may come on most days and last most of the day. Often the patient does not sleep well, cannot pay attention to any one thing, and is tired or dizzy or frightened, or feels very sad (see also Unit 42).

(2) *Some other headaches, called migraine,* last usually only 1–2 days. They can be very painful and they usually come back every few weeks or months. They often start on one side only. During the headache the patient may feel sick, may vomit, does not like to look at bright light, and may have trouble in seeing. Often, the patient knows that the headache is coming in a short time.

First, explain to the patient that there is no serious disease in the head. If the patient has not tried treatment with aspirin before, give aspirin before or at the beginning of the headache. If it helps, the patient should take aspirin each time to prevent or reduce the headache.

Sometimes you and the patient can find out whether this headache seems to come after the patient has taken certain foods or drinks.

In that case, the patient should avoid those foods. Often, the only useful treatment is rest and sleep.

Headaches that may be a sign of a serious disease

The patient has a headache for the first time and it began last week

Find out:

- if the patient has fever (see Unit 24)
- if his neck is stiff.

To find out if the neck is stiff:

- lay the patient on his back
- put your hand under his neck
- try to lift his head.

If the neck bends forward (see picture 1), the neck is not stiff.

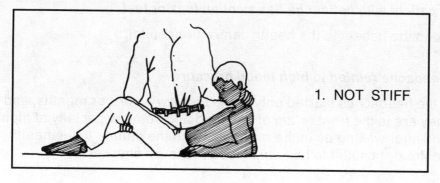

1. NOT STIFF

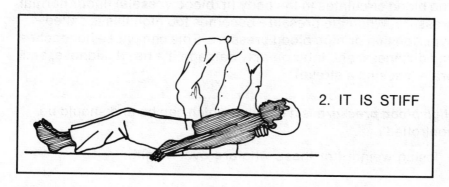

2. IT IS STIFF

If the neck does not bend (see picture 2), it is stiff.

If the patient has a stiff neck, with or without a fever, give him penicillin (procaine benzylpenicillin or ampicillin) as indicated in Annex 1 and give him something to drink. Then send him to the hospital if it is not too far away. If the hospital is too far away, survey the patient and continue the penicillin. If you have no penicillin, you can give sulfamethoxazole + trimethoprim as indicated in Annex 1.

A woman has headache and is more than 5 months pregnant.

Send her to the health centre or hospital.

A patient has a headache and has also started behaving strangely.

See Unit 42, "Mental health and mental disorders".

A patient with headache has swollen legs or feet.

Send the patient to the health centre or hospital.

Headache related to high blood pressure

If the headaches started only in the last few weeks or months, and they are in the front or top of the head and come especially at night and after waking up in the morning, send the patient to the health centre or hospital to have his blood pressure checked.

The blood circulates in the body (in blood vessels) under normal pressure. When the pressure becomes too high this is called hypertension or high blood pressure. This can cause headaches and dizziness, and later on may damage the heart, kidneys, and brain (causing a stroke).

High blood pressure is a disease which can be and should be controlled by:

■ losing weight (for those who are overweight);

- reducing (or avoiding) salt in the diet;
- taking special medicines (ask your supervisor).

When such medicines are given to your patients you should check from time to time that the patients are taking them regularly.

Belly pains

Most belly pains are linked to diarrhoea, constipation, intestinal worms, or menstruation, and can be treated in the community without the patient having to go to the hospital.

When a belly pain is severe and is gradually getting worse and the patient looks ill, then this can be very serious. The patient must be taken to hospital at once.

Learning objectives

After studying this unit you should be able to:

1 Advise what to do when a patient has sudden and severe pain in the belly

- for the first time
- not for the first time.

2 Treat and advise a patient who has pains in the belly from time to time.

What to do

When you see a patient who has belly pains, you should ask
whether the pain is very bad or not and whether it is the first time
that it has happened.

When the pain is very severe

- Did the pain start a few minutes or a few hours ago?
- Is it very bad and getting worse?
- Is the patient vomiting?
- Is he constipated, or feeling sick?
- Is the belly swollen and hard and tender to the touch?

(1) If it is the first time that the patient has felt this pain, you should
take or send the patient to the hospital immediately. He should not
eat or drink anything.

(2) If it is not the first time that the patient has felt this pain, and
the pain comes and goes (there may or may not be diarrhoea), give

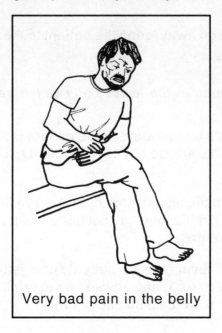

Very bad pain in the belly

the patient aluminium hydroxide (see Annex 1) and ask him to lie down for 2 hours. See him again after 2 hours. If the pain has gone, let the patient go home and tell him to come back if the pain starts again. If the pain continues or starts again, send him to the hospital or health centre.

When the pain is not very bad

(1) If the patient has diarrhoea, see Unit 26.

(2) If the patient has worms in the faeces, see Unit 38.

The patient has pain which usually comes about 2 hours after a meal

Advise the patient not to eat fatty foods (fried food, cakes), to eat slowly, and to rest for half an hour after eating. Give aluminium hydroxide (see Annex 1). See the patient again after 2 weeks.

If the pain has gone, stop the treatment, but advise him again to avoid fatty foods, and to eat slowly. Advise him also to return to see you in a week.

If the pain does not go away, send the patient to the health centre or hospital.

The patient has pains in the lower belly which get worse when he urinates

(1) Take the patient's temperature. If the patient is not feverish give aspirin (see Annex 1). Advise him to drink plenty of fluids. See him again after 3 days.

If there is no more pain, advise him to drink more fluids than usual for a few more days. If the pain has not gone, send him to the hospital or health centre.

(2) If the patient has fever give the patient sulfamethoxazole + trimethoprim (see Annex 1) and advise him to drink more fluids than usual. See the patient again after 5 days.

If there is no more pain or fever, the patient is probably cured. Advise him to drink more fluids than usual for a few more days. If he does not get better, send him to the hospital or health centre.

Belly pains in women

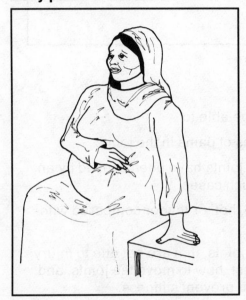

(1) *A woman has belly pains every time she has her period.* See Unit 19.

(2) *A pregnant woman has pains in the belly*. See Unit 15.

Belly pains in an old man

If the patient is an old man (over 55 years of age) who has pain while urinating, and who urinates very often, see Unit 13. Send this person to the hospital.

Unit 29

Pains in joints, back, and neck

Many people have pains in the joints of the arms or legs, or in the back and neck. These pains make it hard for them to do their normal daily work. They need care to relieve the pains. They also need to keep their joints as active as possible by moving them.

Learning objectives

After studying this unit you should be able to:

1 Explain to people the main causes of pains in the joints.

2 Find out whether the pains in the joints have been caused by an injury and advise what to do in such cases.

3 Decide whether a joint is swollen, hot, or tender compared with other joints.

4 Advise persons with pains in the joints, that are not due to injury, how to relieve the pain, how to rest, how to move the joints, and how to keep the muscles strong to prevent stiffness.

5 Make a bandage of cloth to support the ankle and wrist joints.

6 Decide when an adult or a child with one or several painful joints should be sent to the hospital or health centre.

7 Explain to people the main causes of pains in the back and neck.

8 Advise persons how to relieve pains in the back, neck and shoulders, and how to prevent such pains.

What causes pains in the joints

Pains in the joints can be caused by:

- injury
- infection with germs and other diseases of joints (causing swollen and hot joints)
- old age (causing changes in the joints).

Pains caused by an injury

An accident may have injured one or several joints.

(1) *There is a wound.* See Unit 31 "Wounds" on page 247.

(2) *There is a broken bone.* See Unit 33 "Fractures" on page 260.

(3) *There is a sprain.* A sprain is a severe twisting of a joint, often the ankle. It causes swelling of the area around the joint. Put a bandage around the joint to hold it firm (see drawing). This will reduce pain due to movement. The bandage should neither be too tight nor too loose. If the bandage is too tight it will cause pain or swelling below the joint (in the toes). If this happens, the bandage should be taken off and applied less tightly. The patient should rest the injured part. If there is a lot of pain, give aspirin tablets (see Annex 1). See the patient again in 3 days.

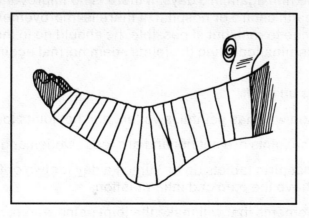

- If the swelling and pain are much less, tell the patient to rest the foot for another 3–4 days.
- If there is no improvement, send the patient to the health centre or hospital.

Examining the painful joints

Compare the painful joint with the same joint on the other side of the body.

- Is the joint swollen?

Gently place your hand on the joint:

- Is it hot? Does pressure cause more pain?

Joint pains not caused by injuries

The patient is a young person or a child

When you find that one or more joints are painful, swollen, and hot, ask the patient if he recently had a sore throat or diarrhoea.

If yes, send him to the health centre or hospital (he should not walk). If not, advise him to rest until there is no more pain or swelling and give aspirin (see dosage for children and adults in Annex 1). See him again in 3 days. If there is no improvement send him to the health centre or hospital. If there is improvement, he should continue to rest, but, if possible, he should go to the health centre for examination when the joints seem normal again.

The patient is an adult

Tell the person who has painful, swollen, and hot joints to:

- rest until the joints are not hot and are less swollen and painful
- take 1 or 2 aspirin tablets up to 3 times a day for two or three days to relieve the pain and inflammation
- avoid movements that will make the joint pains worse, but to change position often to relieve pain and stiffness

■ move the joints as far as they will go in each direction without causing pain, several times a day, to prevent stiffness.

In this way the person will be able to use the joints fully when the pain and swelling go away. If the joints are moved regularly the muscles around the joints do not lose their strength.

See the patient again after 3 days. If there is no improvement send the person to the health centre or hospital.

The person is an old man or woman

In old people the painful joints are not usually hot or swollen, but they are stiff after rest and sleep. The stiffness is relieved by gentle movements but the stiffness and pain get worse after physical exercise such as a long walk. Joint pains at night are common.

Give aspirin (see Annex 1) when the person cannot sleep or when pains are severe after physical exercise.

General advice for persons with pains in the joints

When the hips and knees are painful

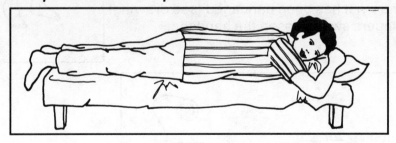

Advise the patient to:

■ rest lying flat on the stomach with the feet over the edge of the bed so that the hips and knee joints can be kept straight (see drawing above)

■ lie down flat, stand up or walk, and not to sit or crouch for a long time

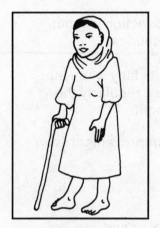

■ use a walking stick; if the hip or knee on one side only is affected, the patient should hold the stick in the hand on the side opposite to that of the pain.

Joint pains in the arms and hands

Ask the patient to use both arms when lifting things (see drawing) and climb a stool or a ladder to lift things to high places.

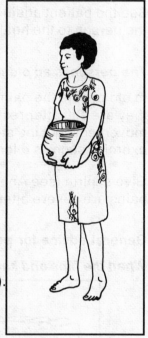

When the wrist is very painful it should be bandaged to hold it firm; this will reduce the pain. Full movement must be possible in the thumb and fingers. The fingers must not swell after the wrist has been bandaged (see drawing). If the fingers swell, loosen the bandage.

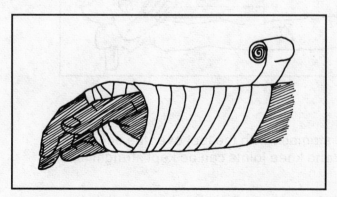

A person with painful wrists who cannot easily use a spoon or knife for cooking or eating should cover their handles with a thick material such as rubber or bamboo (see drawing). This should make it less painful to hold the utensils.

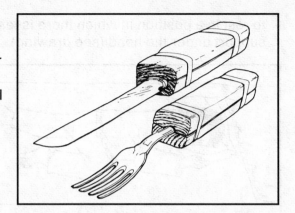

Pain in the back

Back pain can be caused by:

- injury during exercise or work
- lifting or carrying heavy objects incorrectly
- unsuitable positions of the body, such as twisting or bending forward for a long time.

Advice for persons with sudden pain in the back

The pain will be less if such people:

- lie or sleep in a position that eases the pain
- take aspirin (see Annex 1)
- do not lift or carry heavy objects
- avoid walking on uneven ground, or up or down hill
- do not sit, but stand or lie down.

General advice for persons with back pain

Ask such patients:

- not to make movements that are painful, and especially not to twist the body during lifting

■ to rest in a position in which there is less pain and with a low support under the head (see drawing)

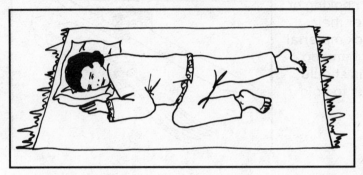

■ to bend the knees when lifting any object or a child from the ground, and to hold the lifted object close to the body (see drawing).

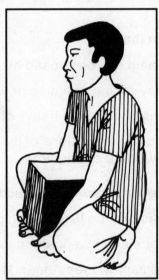

Pains in the neck and shoulders

Such pains are caused by:

■ working with the arms raised for a long time

■ working or sitting or standing with the arms, head, and neck in the same position for a long time

■ twisting the neck

■ injury to the head or shoulders

■ old age (changes in the neck and shoulders).

Advice for persons with pains in the neck and shoulders

Ask the patient to:

- avoid movements and positions that will make the pain worse

- change working position and rest hands and arms as often as possible

- stretch and move the back, head, and shoulders regularly so as to prevent pain or stiffness, if the person must sit or stand in one position while working

- have gentle massage over neck and shoulder muscles, if this relieves pain

- take aspirin, if the person cannot sleep or when pains are severe

- use a loose collar of folded towel or cloth around the neck to give support under the chin so as to relieve pain (see drawing).

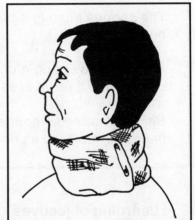

Important!

Remember that aspirin is an effective, cheap, and easily available drug to relieve pains in the joints and in the back.

Unit 30

Burns

Burns are caused by:

- fire
- hot or burning objects
- boiling water or oil (burns are then called "scalds")
- electric shock
- some chemicals (such as acids and alkalis).

The serious thing in a burn is the area of the skin that is burned.

A burn is always painful. It may be dangerous and cause death when a large area of the skin is burned.

Before treating someone who has been burned, wash your hands carefully so as not to get germs in the burn.

Learning objectives

After studying this unit you should be able to:

1 Tell whether a burn covers a small or a large area of the skin.

2 Tell when a patient with burns should be sent to the hospital or health centre.

3 Decide what to do when a large area of the skin is burned.

4 Take care of patients who only have a small area of the skin burned:

- when they come less than 24 hours after the burn
- when they come more than 24 hours after the burn.

5 Decide what to do in the case of chemical burns of the skin.

6 Discuss with the community and suggest measures to prevent burns.

242

How much skin has been burned?

A large area has been burned when the burn covers as much as the whole of one arm, or the whole of one leg, or the head, or half the back, or more than half the chest. When it is less than that, the burn is said to cover a small area of the skin.

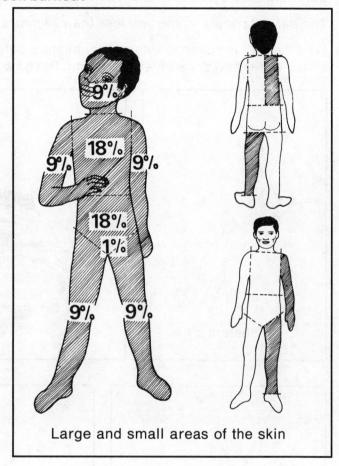

Large and small areas of the skin

If a large area of the skin is burned

Send the patient to the hospital or health centre immediately, but first:

- lay the patient on a stretcher
- cover the burned part with a clean cloth
- give plenty of water to drink
- if possible, give an injection of penicillin in the buttock (see Annex 2).

If a small area of the skin is burned

The patient comes to see you less than 24 hours after the burn

(1) If the skin is covered with watery blisters only, wash gently with soapy water and dry with a clean cloth. Put on a loose dressing

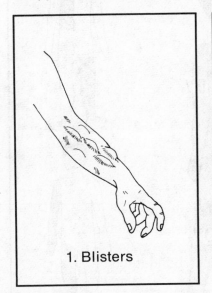

1. Blisters

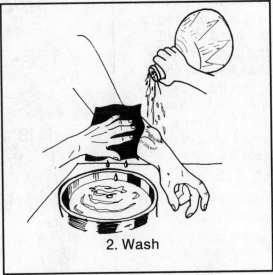

2. Wash

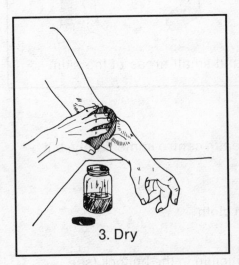

3. Dry

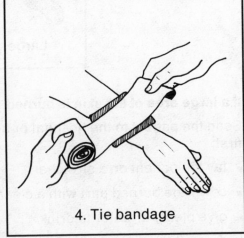

4. Tie bandage

(see drawing). Tell the patient not to take the bandage off or to dirty it. Take the dressing off after a week.

■ If the skin smells bad, or if there is a discharge, see paragraph (2) below.

■ If the skin does not smell bad and is dry, leave it uncovered. The patient will get better without any further treatment.

(2) If the skin is covered in blood, or in yellow fluid, wash gently with warm salty water and a clean cloth. If the burn is on an arm or a leg, place the burned limb on a clean cloth soaked in warm salty water. Leave the burned area uncovered but ask the patient to keep flies away from the burned skin. When available, give an injection of tetanus antitoxin (serum) (see Annex 1). Then give an injection of procaine benzylpenicillin every day for 5 days (see Annex 1). If you have no procaine benzylpenicillin, give sulfamethoxazole + trimethoprim tablets (see Annex 1). The patient must drink plenty of water while taking these tablets. Repeat the care of the skin (as above) every 2 days until a thin scab covers the wound. Then put on a loose bandage (see drawing no. 4). If the patient becomes feverish at any time, send him to the hospital or health centre.

The patient comes to see you more than 24 hours after the burn

Wash the skin with warm water and soap, gently trying to rub off any dirt with a clean cloth until the skin starts bleeding a little.

Then follow the instructions in paragraph (2) above.

Chemical burn of the skin

This is an emergency. You should immediately wash away the chemical with large amounts of water for several minutes. Then do as for other burns (see above).

Always be careful not to get any of the chemical on yourself.

How to prevent burns

Discuss with the people in the community how to prevent burns,
for instance by:

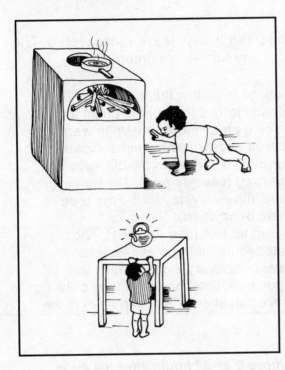

- raising stoves or fires
  half a metre from the
  ground so that children
  cannot reach them

- putting a guard around a
  fire

- keeping hot water, fires,
  matches, and chemicals
  out of the reach of
  children

- having no bare electric
  wires in the house

- advising women not to
  wear clothes made from
  synthetic material when
  they are cooking food on
  an open fire.

Remember!

*It is mainly women and children who get burned. Women may
get burned when they cook food on a fire, and children get
burned because they do not realize the danger.*

*Remind parents and older children how they can protect
young children from these dangers.*

Never put butter, fat, grease, herbs or dirt on any burn.

Unit 31

Wounds

A wound is a cut or a tear in the skin.

All wounds bleed, are painful, and can easily become infected. Some may hide a fracture or internal bleeding. They may also lead to shock.

A wound should be carefully cleaned and then protected with a bandage or a clean cloth.

Learning objectives

After studying this unit you should be able to:

1 Examine a wounded person.

2 Give first aid to stop bleeding.

3 Take action if there is a broken bone.

4 Decide what to do if there is shock.

5 Treat and dress wounds.

6 Treat infected wounds.

247

Examining the wounded person

First look at the person

- Is he conscious?
- Is he very pale?

To find out if there are any other injuries, other than the ones you can see, ask him, or people with him, what happened, and when and how it happened.

Look at the wound itself and ask yourself:

- Is the patient losing a lot of blood through the wound?
- Is there a broken bone underneath? (see Unit 33)
- Is there shock? (see Unit 32)

The patient is losing a lot of blood through the wound but there is no fracture

You should try to stop the bleeding. Raise the bleeding part above the rest of the body. Press down hard on the wound with a clean cloth to stop the bleeding. Keep pressing for at least 10 minutes, then take the cloth off and see whether the blood is still coming out. If the bleeding has stopped, make the patient drink some water and treat the wound(s).

If the bleeding continues, raise the bleeding part again and tie a tight bandage around the place which is bleeding. If the blood comes through the bandage, tie another bandage around it, tighter than the first one.

See whether the patient is weak and very tired. If the patient is thirsty, give him rehydration fluid (sugar, salt, and water) and send him to the hospital or health centre on a stretcher.

There is a broken bone.

See Unit 33, page 260.

The wound is deep.

Deep wounds are usually caused by gunshots, stabbing, or when a long piece of metal or glass cuts into the body. Deep wounds are dangerous, particularly when they are in the chest or belly.

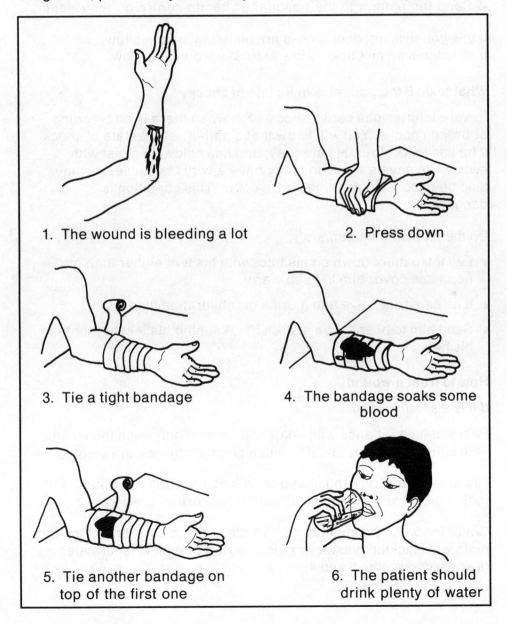

1. The wound is bleeding a lot

2. Press down

3. Tie a tight bandage

4. The bandage soaks some blood

5. Tie another bandage on top of the first one

6. The patient should drink plenty of water

Do the following *immediately*:

- Clean the wound superficially with a clean cloth.
- If possible, tie a bandage to reduce bleeding.
- Send the patient to the hospital or health centre on a stretcher.

If the wound is not deep and is not bleeding much, follow instructions given under "How to treat a wound", below.

What to do if the patient is in a state of shock

Severe injuries can cause shock even when there is no bleeding or broken bones. You will know that a patient is in a state of shock if he has lost colour, is pale grey, and has cold skin moist with sweat. He may be weak and may have a very fast pulse. He may also be unconscious or may be in coma. This condition is dangerous.

Do the following *immediately:*

- Lay the patient down on his back with his feet higher than his head and cover him to keep warm.
- If he can drink, give him a drink of rehydration fluid.
- Send him to hospital on a stretcher, keeping his feet higher than his head.

How to treat a wound

If it is a small wound

First wash your hands with soap and water. Then wash the wound with soap and water, and dry with a clean cloth (see drawing no. 1).

Clean away any dirt and shave off any hair around the wound. Put iodine on the wound and all around it (see drawing no. 2).

Cover the wound completely with a clean piece of cloth. Fasten the cloth with sticking plaster or pins or string or a piece of creeper (see drawings nos. 3 and 4).

Tell the patient not to dirty the bandage or to take it off. Give an injection of tetanus antitoxin (serum) (see Annex 1).

Take the bandage off after 2 days and put on a new one. Change the bandage every 2 days until the wound has healed and become dry.

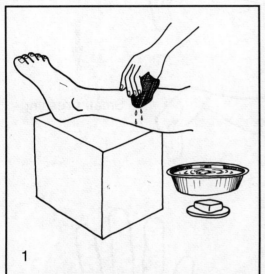

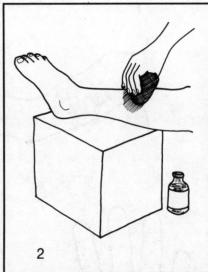

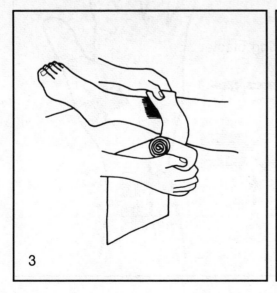

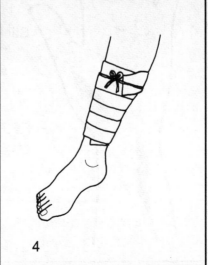

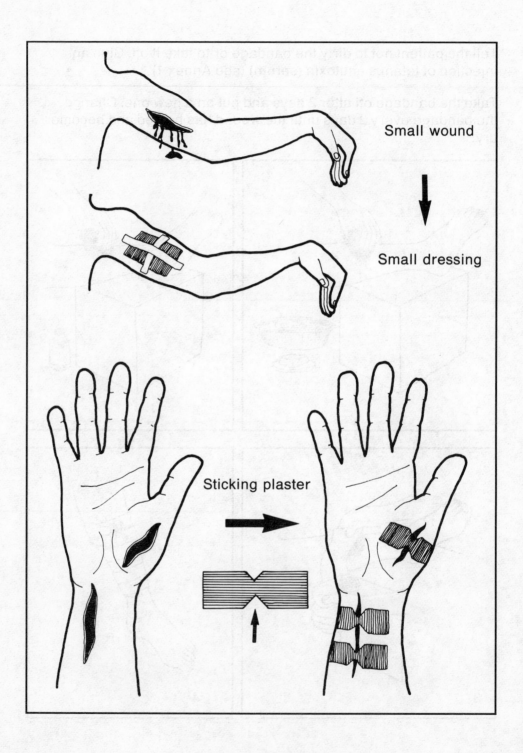

Small wound

Small dressing

Sticking plaster

252

How to dress a wound on the head

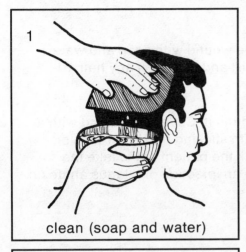

1

clean (soap and water)

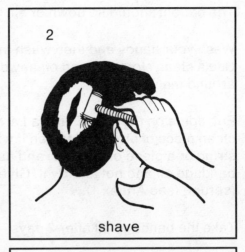

2

shave

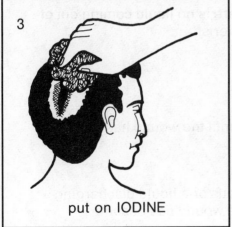

3

put on IODINE

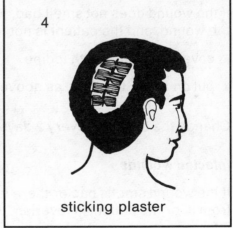

4

sticking plaster

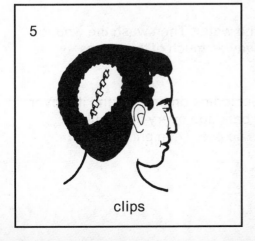

5

clips

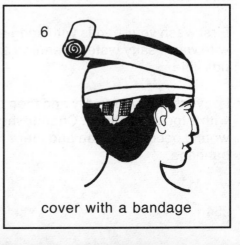

6

cover with a bandage

If it is a large wound (over 5 cm long)

The patient should lie down or sit.

Wash your hands and then wash the wound with soap and water. Use a clean cloth to clean off any dirt and shave off any hair around the wound.

Put iodine on the wound and all around it. Cover the wound with a clean piece of cloth and fasten it with sticking plaster or pins or string or a piece of creeper, and ask the patient not to take the bandage off and not to dirty it. Give an injection of tetanus antitoxin (serum) (see Annex 1).

Take the bandage off after 2 days.

If the wound does not smell bad, there is no liquid coming out of the wound, and the patient is not feverish:

- cover the wound with iodine

- put on a new bandage as above.

Change the bandage every 2 days until the wound has healed.

Infected wounds.

If the wound smells bad or there is pus or a liquid discharging from it, or the patient is feverish, the wound has become infected.

First wash your hands with soap and water. Then wash the wound with warm salty water, cleaning away as much of the pus as possible.

Leave the wound to dry and then put iodine on and around it. Cover with a loose bandage. Change the bandage every day until the wound becomes clean and there is no pus. Then put on a new bandage.

Give the patient one injection of procaine benzylpenicillin every day for 3 days:

- *children*:   500 000 units
- *adults*:   1 000 000 units.

If you have no procaine benzylpenicillin, give sulfamethoxazole + trimethoprim tablets;

- *children*: 1 tablet, morning, noon, and night for 3 days
- *adults*:   2 tablets, 4 times a day for 3 days.

If after a week the wound still smells bad, if there is still some liquid coming out of the wound, or if the patient is still feverish, send the patient to the health centre or hospital

---

Remember!

Always wash your hands with water and soap before and after treating a wound.

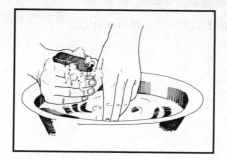

Unit 32
Bleeding and shock

Bleeding can be very dangerous. When you see a person who is bleeding, you must try to stop it as quickly as possible. You will often need to take or send the patient to the health centre.

The blood carries oxygen from the lungs to every part of the body. If the body loses too much blood it cannot get enough oxygen, and without oxygen the person will die.

When a person is in a state of shock, he feels weak, becomes unconscious, and is pale and cold with a very fast and weak pulse. Shock may be due to severe bleeding, an accident, a blow, a wound, severe burns, diarrhoea, or vomiting.

Learning objectives

After studying this unit you should be able to:

1 Identify where the bleeding you can see is coming from, provide first aid, and advise the patient what to do.

2 Tell what signs make you suspect that a patient is bleeding inside his body and advise what to do.

3 Deal with a patient suffering from shock.

Bleeding from different parts of the body and what to do about it

There are two types of bleeding: one that you can see (bleeding outside the body), and one that you cannot see (bleeding inside the body). Both need urgent action.

Bleeding from a wound that has cut the skin or from an open fracture.

See Units 31 and 33 for instructions on how to treat wounds and fractures respectively.

Vomiting of dark brown blood (*like coffee*)

If the patient vomits blood that is dark brown in colour, it probably comes from his stomach. The patient should not eat or drink anything and should be sent to hospital at once.

Coughing up blood

The patient coughs up red blood. There may be enough blood to fill a cup or there may be only a little blood mixed with sputum. The blood probably comes from the lungs. Tell your patient to rest, and arrange to have him taken to the hospital at once (see also Unit 11, "Tuberculosis").

Bleeding through the vagina

If the woman is pregnant, see Unit 15.

If the woman is not pregnant, see Unit 19.

Bleeding through the anus

If the patient has been passing black blood mixed with faeces for several days, he may be feeling weak and dizzy. The blood is coming from the stomach or gut.

The patient should go to the hospital or health centre without delay.

Bleeding from the nose

The person should sit down but should not lie down. He should pinch his nose with his fingers for 15 minutes or put cotton wool in his nose. He should not blow his nose for at least an hour.

Bleeding from an ear

If this happens after an accident or a blow on the head, the patient is in danger. It may be that the brain is injured. Do not put anything into the ear. The patient should lie down with the head bent towards the ear which is bleeding. He should be carried to the health centre or hospital at once.

How to tell when there is bleeding inside the body and what to do

Sometimes a person bleeds heavily inside the body but the blood does not come out. You should suspect this when an injury is caused by an accident, a blow, a kick, a bullet, or knife.

A patient who is bleeding inside the body feels weak or faints (becomes unconscious). Try to take his pulse (see "Counting the pulse" in Annex 2). It will be very fast and weak. The skin will be pale, cold, and damp (cold sweat). *This is shock.* It is very dangerous.

Lie the patient down on his back with the feet higher than the head, and cover him to keep him warm. Give him some rehydration fluid if he is able to drink. Then send him to hospital immediately on a stretcher.

If the bleeding is inside the head the patient will become unconscious and may die if he is not treated in hospital.

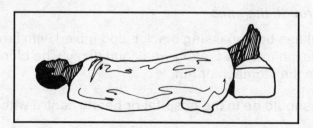

Sometimes a woman in early pregnancy may have heavy bleeding inside the body. She will have severe pain in the lower belly (see Unit 19).

Remember!

After an accident you should examine the whole body to find out if there are any hidden wounds under the patient's clothes. Also look for signs of internal bleeding.

Be careful when carrying a wounded person. If you lift him in the wrong way you may make his injury worse (see Units 31 and 33).

Unit 33
Fractures

When a bone is broken it is called a fracture.

Fractures are treated in different ways depending on which bone is broken.

All patients who have a suspected fracture must be sent to the health centre or hospital for final diagnosis and proper treatment.

Great care must be taken when carrying a patient with a broken bone. If he is carried in the wrong way his injury may become worse.

Learning objectives

After studying this unit you should be able to:

1 Find out whether there is a fracture and say where you suspect the fracture is.

2 Find out whether there is any other injury to the body (such as a wound or another fracture).

3 Do what is necessary in each case.

4 Send the patient to the hospital or health centre, making sure that the injury will not get worse in the meantime.

How to tell if there is a fracture

If a person has had a fall or a violent blow, there is probably a broken bone in a limb if:

- it hurts a lot when the patient tries to move the injured limb
- the patient is not able to move the limb at all
- it hurts a lot when you press gently the injured part
- there is a change in the shape of the limb at the place where there is pain.

There is a broken bone if:

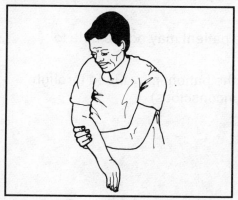

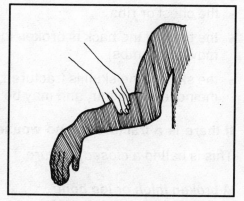

- it hurts a lot when the patient tries to move the injured limb

- it hurts when you press the injured part

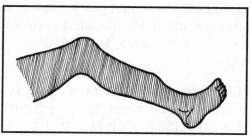

- there is a change in the shape of the limb at the place where there is pain

261

What to do in case of a fracture

Do not move the bone that may be broken because this will cause severe pain and may make the fracture worse and cause bleeding.

First, see whether there is a wound in addition to the fracture. If there is, you should treat the wound first.

Examine the rest of the body in case there is another fracture or wound. Is another limb out of shape? More than one bone may be broken.

Is there a bad pain somewhere else? For example, in:

- the pelvis
- the chest or ribs
- the back (if the back is broken the patient may not be able to move any limbs)
- the skull (if the skull is fractured, the patient may bleed through the nose or the ear, and may be unconscious).

If there is a fracture but no wound

This is called a *closed fracture.*

A broken thigh or leg bone

Give aspirin tablets for the pain (see Annex 1).

Splint the whole of both legs. A broken thigh or leg will be kept from moving by tying both the legs together at 4 or more points with sufficient padding (cotton, towels, etc.) between the legs at the upper thighs, the knees, the ankles, and the feet so that they cannot move (see drawing no. 1).

However, do not tie the legs together if the pelvis is injured. In that case, support the two limbs on a wooden board and raise them slightly above the level of the body (see drawing no. 2). Send the patient to the hospital or health centre, strapped to a wooden board or stretcher. He may drink water if he wishes to, but he should not eat if he is going to hospital in case he has to have an operation.

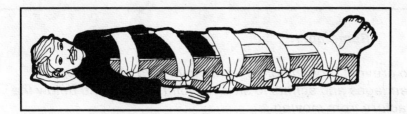

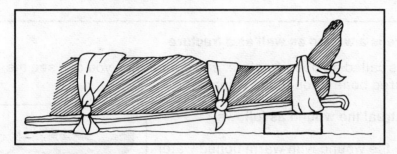

A broken arm or forearm

Give aspirin tablets for the pain (see Annex 1).
Put the arm in a sling and fix it to the chest with a bandage round the chest so that the broken arm cannot move (see drawing) and send the patient to the hospital.

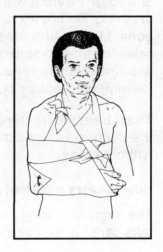

Another part of the body is broken (ribs, back, pelvis, head)

Give aspirin tablets for pain (see Annex 1). Send the patient to the hospital on a hard stretcher.

Remember!

To prevent broken bones from moving you should use bandages and splints to stop the joints above and below the fracture from moving.

If there is a wound as well as a fracture

This is called an *open fracture*, and sometimes you can see the fractured bone through the wound.

First, treat the wound as follows:

Clean the wound with warm boiled water and soap. Cover it with a very clean dressing. Do not try to push back the bone. Make a firm pressure bandage and raise the limb to stop or decrease the bleeding (see Unit 32). Give aspirin tablets to relieve pain. Give an injection of tetanus antitoxin (serum) (see Annex 1).

Then, treat the fracture as described above depending on where the fracture is. Send the patient to the hospital or health centre without delay.

How to carry a patient properly

The important thing to remember is to take care not to make the injury worse.

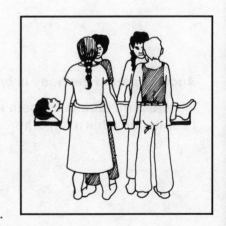

When an arm is broken, put it in a sling fixed to the chest (see page 263). The patient may walk and sit.

When a thigh or leg is broken, the patient should not be moved before a splint has been put on the injured limb. The patient should be carried on a hard stretcher. This may be a board or a door.

When you think there may be an injury to the back, neck, chest, or pelvis, do not try to move the patient until you have at least three other people to help you. Then get a board (a stretcher or door) quickly. With the help of the other people lie the patient on the board. **Do not move the patient more than is necessary to put him on the board.** Also, make sure the board is wide enough and at least as long as the patient's height.

Then, carefully carry the board with the patient to the health centre or hospital.

Further care of the patient

If the patient stays at home or returns from the hospital you should see him again within 24 hours. See whether he has pain, whether the fingers or toes are blue or cold, and whether he is unable to move the toes or fingers. If you find any of these things, the patient should go to the hospital at once.

Unit 34

Bites

All animal bites can be dangerous and may cause death. They should be treated as quickly as possible.

All bites (and wounds) carry the danger of infection, especially tetanus, and should be thoroughly cleaned (see Unit 31).

Some initial bleeding is not serious: it can even help in bringing out the germs of infection.

Snake bites are always dangerous, but fortunately they are not always fatal.

There is usually somebody in the community who knows how to treat snake bites with local methods. You should talk with these people; they may be able to help if you have no antivenom.

Learning objectives

After studying this unit you should be able to:

1 Treat a wound caused by a dog bite.

2 Identify signs in a dog's behaviour that mean that the dog is acting strangely and might have rabies.

3 Treat a person who has been bitten by a snake.

A person has been bitten by a dog

Treat the person who has been bitten as follows:

- Clean the wound thoroughly with soap and water.

- Then put iodine on and around the wound with a cloth or cotton wool.

- Bandage the bitten area.

- Give an injection of tetanus antitoxin (serum) if you have some (see Annex 1).

- *Do not* put sticking plaster on the wound.

Find out whether someone knows the dog that bit the patient

Somone knows the dog. If it is the family dog or a neighbour's dog, find out whether the dog's behaviour has changed recently:

- has it stopped eating?

- does it bark in an unusual way?

- does it tremble, behave savagely, bark continuously?

- has it had convulsions (fits)?

- does saliva run out of its mouth?

If the dog showed any of these signs it might have rabies. The dog must be killed and the patient must be sent to the hospital or health centre *at once*. If possible, send the killed dog with the patient for examination.

If the dog shows none of these signs, ask the family of the patient to watch the dog for ten days. If the dog begins to show any of the above signs, it must be killed and the patient must be sent to the hospital or health centre *at once*. If the dog stays healthy, you need do nothing else.

No one knows the dog. If the dog does not belong to the community, send the patient to the health centre or hospital.

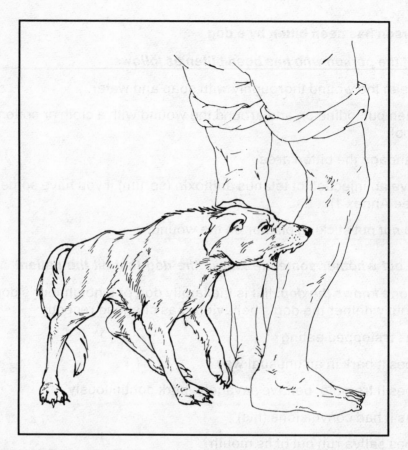

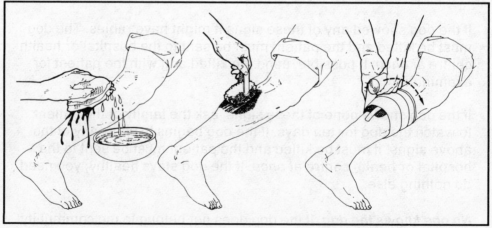

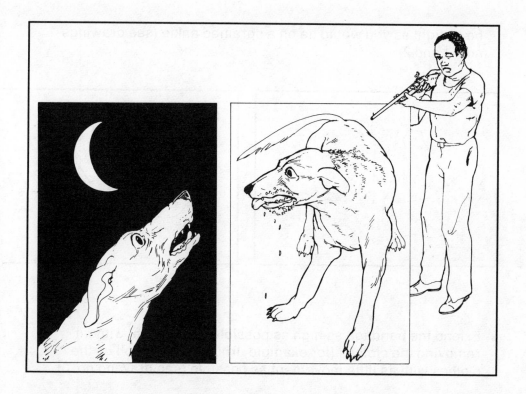

A person has been bitten by a snake

Explain to the patient and the family that many snake bites, even those of poisonous snakes, do not cause death, and that the patient can be treated and that they should stay calm.

Calm, rest, and no alcohol will help to slow down the spread of the poison to the rest of the body. Fear and excitement will make the patient worse.

- Clean the wound quickly with soap and water and paint it with iodine.

- Order transport to take the person to the hospital or health centre immediately, where he can be given an injection of antivenom (see Annex 1).

- Meanwhile, tie a broad bandage tightly over the bite as soon as possible. Try not to move the bitten limb. The bandage should

269

be as tight as you would tie on a sprained ankle (see drawings nos. 1 and 2).

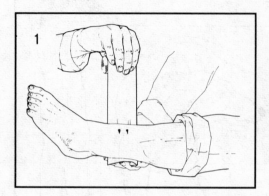
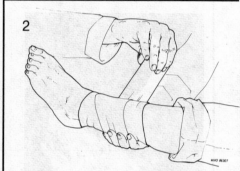

■ Extend the bandage as high as possible on the limb, without removing the clothes (for example, trousers). Just roll up the clothes with as little movement as possible (see drawing no. 3).

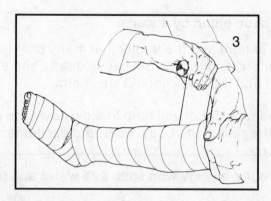

■ Now apply a splint on the limb just as you would do in case of a fracture (see Unit 33). Bind the splint as firmly as possible to the limb (see drawings nos. 4, 5, and 6).

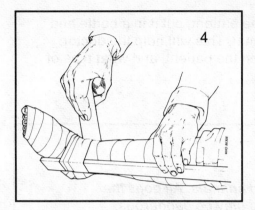

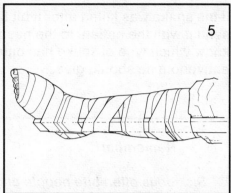

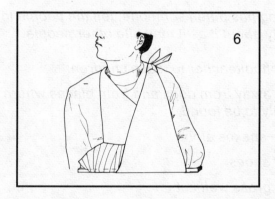

Remember!

- *The bitten limb should be kept as still as possible when you are tying the bandage and splint.*

- *If you tie the bandage and splint correctly, they will be comfortable for several hours. This should give you enough time to take the patient to the hospital.*

- *The bandages and splint should not be taken off until the patient has reached the hospital. Only the doctor can decide when it is safe to remove them.*

If the snake was killed after it bit the patient, put it in a bottle and send it with the patient to the hospital. This will help the doctor know which type of snake has bitten the patient, and what type of antivenom he should give.

Remember!

Sick dogs often bite people and animals. All dogs that wander around the countryside may be dangerous.

If a sick dog has bitten someone, tell the people in the community about it as it may bite other people.

Ask the schoolteacher to teach children:

- *to keep away from dogs and from places where snakes are likely to be found*
- *to leave snakes alone*
- *to wear shoes*
- *to keep grass well cut*
- *to use a torch when walking around at night.*

Unit 35

Poisoning

Poisoning is common in children, mainly between the ages of one and four years.

Adults take poison, sometimes deliberately and sometimes by accident.

Poisoning can be prevented.

Learning objectives

After studying this unit you should be able to:

1 Identify the common poisonous substances in the community and in the neighbourhood.

2 Suspect and recognize acute poisoning.

3 Decide what to do with a patient with acute poisoning.

4 Discuss with the community and suggest ways and means of preventing common poisoning.

Poisonous substances

There are many poisonous substances in houses and their surroundings. In towns and cities, most poisonings in children occur when they drink kerosene thinking it is water. In villages, poisonous seeds and pesticides are the commonest cause. The common poisons are as follows:

In villages	*In cities*
Poisonous seeds	Kerosene
Berries, wild fruit and mushrooms	Drugs and chemicals, such as aspirin,
Pesticides and insecticides	iron tablets, barbiturates, potassium
Kerosene	permanganate
Drugs, e.g., aspirin, chloroquine	Insecticides
	Rat poison

Alcohol and drugs are poisons for adults as well as for children. They are dangerous when taken in excess at any one time (acute poisoning), but also when taken regularly over a long time. Tobacco is also a poison when smoked regularly over a long period of time.

Signs of acute poisoning

There are many signs of acute poisoning (which are the same in adults as in children), for example:

- burns on the lips, and in the mouth and throat, caused by chemicals

- vomiting and diarrhoea

- paralysis (person is unable to move)

- being semi-conscious or unconscious

- being unable to breathe.

If a child who is usually healthy has one or more of these signs, you should think of poisoning. Sometimes the child or another person who was present when the poisoning occurred may be able to tell you or show you what the child had eaten or drunk. If the poisonous substance can be found, you can then be sure that the child is poisoned. Also, the treatment will be easier if the cause is known.

What to do in a case of acute poisoning

If the patient is conscious and has no burns on the lips or in the mouth

First, try at once to make the patient vomit. Do this as follows:

Ask the patient to lie on his belly, with the head lower than the chest. Touch, or ask him to touch, the back of his throat with a finger or a spoon.

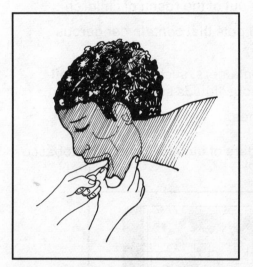 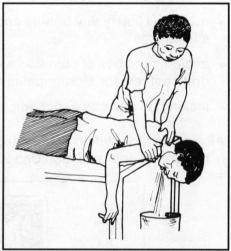

If this does not cause vomiting, give 2 teaspoons of salt in a glass (250 ml) of water, *or* give syrup of ipecacuanha (see Annex 1) 5 ml (or one teaspoon) in 20 ml (or one tablespoon) of clean water. This medicine can be repeated after 15 minutes.

Then, after the patient has finished vomiting give him plenty of clean water or tea to drink. It will help also if you can give him activated charcoal powder (1–2 tablespoons in water, see Annex 1), or the white of a raw egg, or some milk.

If the patient is unconscious and has burns on the lips or in the mouth

Do *not* try to make the patient vomit and do *not* try to give him anything to drink.

Send him to the health centre or hospital at once with some of the poison he has taken.

How to prevent poisoning

Remind the people in your community (women, parents, community committee members, schoolteachers, shopkeepers, etc.) that most cases of poisoning can be prevented, by:

- keeping dangerous substances out of the reach of children

- marking clearly any bottles and pots that contain dangerous substances

- avoiding the use of common containers, such as popular soft-drink bottles, for storing poisonous liquids such as kerosene

- locking up poisons and medicines.

Also, wide advertising of the dangers of alcohol, drugs and tobacco is recommended (see also Unit 22).

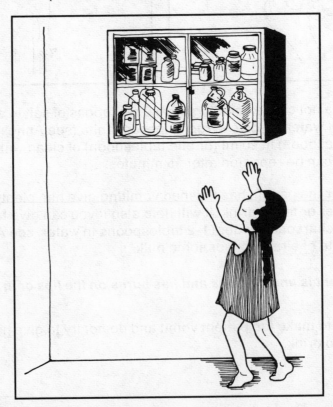

Skin diseases

There are many skin diseases and problems. Only a few of the common and serious skin diseases can be mentioned here.

When there is something wrong with the skin it may be a disease of the skin or a disease of the body that shows on the skin.

Learning objectives

After studying this unit you should be able to:

1 Recognize and treat common skin diseases.

2 Advise families and the community about the care and prevention of common skin diseases.

3 Refer to your supervisor serious skin diseases or diseases of the body that show on the skin.

Causes and signs of skin diseases

Diseases of the skin can be caused by germs or insects, which attack the skin directly, or by a fungus, which is a tiny plant that grows on the skin and damages it. The skin can be damaged also by injury or burns or chemicals.

The skin may also show signs of diseases in the body, for example:

Disease	Signs on the skin
■ Fever	The skin may become red and hot
■ Measles and chickenpox	There is a rash (spots) on the whole body.
■ Leprosy	Parts of the skin become thick and lose the feeling of touch and pain
■ Kwashiorkor (a disease of underfed children)	There is swelling of the body, the skin changes colour and dark thick patches appear on arms and legs

Impetigo

Usually this is a disease of children. There are sores with yellow crusts, often around the mouth and also elsewhere on the patient's skin. These can spread to other people.

Treatment

- Wash the affected skin gently with clean warm water and soap until the crusts come off.

- Cover the sores with gentian violet (see Annex 1) or, if you have a supply, with neomycin/bacitracin ointment (see Annex 1).

- If a large part of the skin is affected and the patient has fever, give procaine benzylpenicillin (see Annex 1).

> **Remember!**
>
> *The crusts are very infectious. Wash your hands very well after you have touched the skin. The patient should keep away from other children.*

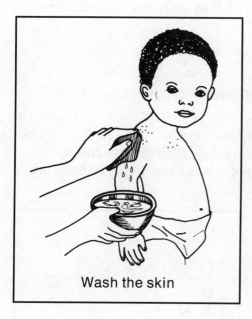

Wash the skin

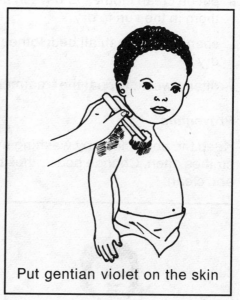

Put gentian violet on the skin

Boils and abscesses

See Unit 41, "Lumps under the skin".

Scabies, or the itch

Very small insects that you cannot see (mites) may make tiny holes in the skin, mostly between the fingers, on the wrists, in front of the elbows, and around the genitals (in young boys). These cause little lumps or blisters that are very itchy. The patient wants to scratch them all the time, and if the finger-nails are long and dirty the scratching can infect the skin and cause sores or small boils.

Treatment

Everybody in the family must be treated at the same time.

Each person must:

- wash the whole body very well with soap and hot water
- cover the whole body with benzyl benzoate (see Annex 1)
- put on clean clothes and wash all clothes worn before and hang them in the sun to dry
- change and wash all bedclothes and hang them in the sun to dry
- after 1 week, repeat the treatment once.

Prevention

Keep the body clean by washing every day. Change into clean clothes often. Change bedclothes often. Keep the finger-nails short and clean.

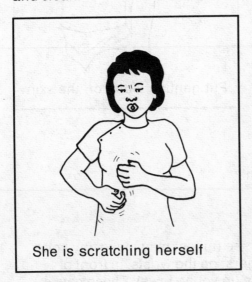

She is scratching herself

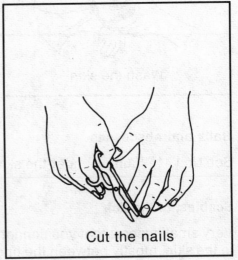

Cut the nails

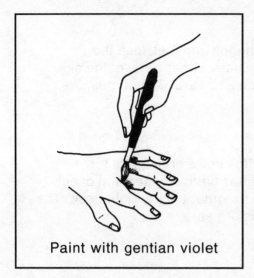

Paint with gentian violet

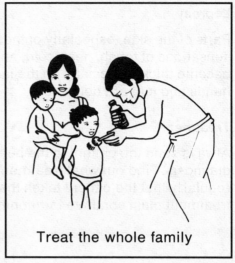

Treat the whole family

Ringworm

The skin shows small rings that grow bigger and itch. On the head the hair falls out in patches. The disease is coming from the finger-nails if they are rough and thick.

Treatment

If the disease is on the scalp, cut the hair short. Wash the itchy areas every day with soap and water. Keep the skin dry and do not cover it. Apply an ointment or cream of benzoic + salicylic acid over the affected parts (see Annex 1).

Keep the finger-nails short and clean. Change underclothes and socks often, and wash them well.

If the disease does not get better in 2–3 weeks send the patient to the health centre.

Prevention

Ringworm spreads easily to other people. The patient should sleep alone and keep away from others until the skin is healed. Follow the general rules of cleanliness.

Leprosy

Parts of the skin, especially of the hands and feet, lose the sensations of touch, heat, cold, and pain. Other parts of the skin become thick, especially on the face and ears. Sometimes, the hands and feet are deformed.

Treatment

Always send the patient to the health centre or hospital for diagnosis. Find out what treatment has been advised and check regularly that the patient takes the treatment in the right dose. The treatment must continue for months or years.

Yaws

If the weather in your country is warm and humid, you may see many cases of yaws. Yaws is mostly a disease of the skin. You will have a special name for the disease in your own language. It spreads easily from one person to another. It usually starts in young children.

The disease shows itself in many ways on the skin. You should learn from your supervisor or from the health centre how it looks in its early stages so that you can treat new cases quickly.

In the beginning there may be one or a few red sores with a yellow top on any part of the body. They may be of any size up to the size of 2 big thumb-nails. They may be dry or moist (slightly wet).

Sometimes in the beginning they are itchy. They spread to other parts of the body by scratching and to other people by direct contact. Sometimes the bone under the skin where there is disease becomes very tender. It hurts a lot when you press it.

The patient is not feverish or sick. Without treatment the sores go away in about 3 months but the germs stay in the body and cause disease later (either the same type of sores or with other signs on the skin and bones).

If your country is in a dry area, you will not find yaws but there may be a disease which is very much like it. It is called endemic syphilis. It also produces red sores with yellow tops, but these sores are dry. Prevention and treatment are the same as for yaws.

Treatment

Remember!

Every patient and every person in a patient's household or in contact with him at school or at work must be treated at the same time.

It is best if a team comes from the health centre so that everybody in a village or community can be treated at the same time. If this cannot be done very soon and you (or your supervisor) have a supply of benzathine benzylpenicillin, treat everyone in the family as follows:

- children between 1 and 10 years of age: one injection of 600 000 units (see Annex 1)

- people over 10 years of age: one injection of 1 200 000 units. This will stop the disease very quickly.

Prevention

Try to tell the people with the disease to keep away from people who do not have it.

The best way to prevent yaws (and most skin diseases) is good personal hygiene: washing properly with water and soap (see Unit 10).

You will learn from your supervisor or the staff of the health centre in your district what is being done to stop yaws in your country or district. Your task in prevention is to inform the health centre about the number of cases of yaws in the community and to help the team that comes to treat all the patients and their contacts.

Remember!

The best way to prevent most skin diseases is good personal hygiene and cleanliness.

Unit 37

Eye diseases and loss of sight

Sight is very precious. People should do everything they can to protect it.

It is very important to prevent and give early treatment for eye diseases and injuries because in many cases they can cause loss of sight.

Children can also become blind from poor nutrition.

The community, with the help of the community health worker, can prevent many eye diseases and loss of sight.

Learning objectives

After studying this unit you should be able to:

1 Find out who are the people with common eye diseases and injuries in your community.

2 Advise people on what they can do to prevent or treat most eye diseases and injuries.

3 Recognize and treat common eye diseases and injuries.

4 Advise which patients should be sent to the health centre or hospital.

Common eye diseases and injuries

First, find out how many people in the community have eye problems, how many cannot see well, and how many are blind. Report your findings to the community leaders or committee and let the committee and the people know that many of these problems can be prevented or treated.

Usually, people get eye diseases because:

■ They rub their eyes with dirty hands or cloths and cause infection.

■ They do not protect their eyes properly while working – for example, when chopping firewood, breaking stones, or harvesting.

■ They do not eat a balanced diet, with plenty of vitamin A, which is found in green leafy vegetables, carrots, and fruits such as papaya and mangoes.

Children sometimes get eye injuries from playing with their toys.

Preventing eye diseases

You should be able to advise members of your community on how to keep good sight and how to prevent blindness.

The best general advice you can give is:

■ People should keep the face and hands clean by washing with soap and water. They should not rub their eyes with the fingers or with a cloth used for drying or cleaning other parts of the body. Since flies can carry eye diseases, they should keep their houses and their surroundings clean to keep down the number of flies.

■ All adults and children should eat a well-balanced diet containing plenty of vitamin A.

■ Birth attendants can prevent red discharging eyes of newborn babies (see page 287).

- Children should learn clean habits at school and should know how to avoid getting eye diseases.
- People should seek early treatment for all eye diseases and injuries and for any loss of sight.

You can also discuss with village leaders, the community committee, and families how eye diseases and blindness are connected with dirt and poor nutrition, and how good nutrition, personal cleanliness, a clean water supply, and good sanitation can keep eyes healthy (see Units 4, 6, and 7).

Some blinding diseases start slowly but may become severe quickly. People should seek advice as soon as they notice that the sight in one or both of their eyes is not as good as it was before.

How to treat common eye diseases

Red discharging eyes in a newborn

When a baby who is only a few days old gets red eyes and there is a discharge of pus from one or both eyes, this is very serious. If it is not treated properly at once, the baby will become blind. The baby has caught an infection in the mother's birth passage while being born. This means that the mother and, probably, the father have one of the diseases spread by sexual contact (see Unit 43).

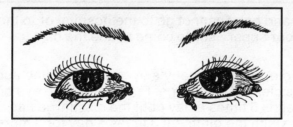

You should send or go with the baby and the parents to the hospital or health centre *at once*. Do not delay.

Treatment. Before the family leave for the hospital or health centre, treat the baby as follows:

- Wash out all discharge from the eyes and clean the eyelids with a clean cloth and water that has been boiled and cooled.

Be careful! The discharge is very infectious. Wash your hands very well afterwards with water and soap.

- Put tetracycline eye ointment under the lids.

- If you have penicillin, give the baby an injection (in the buttock) of 75 000 units of procaine benzylpenicillin (see Annex 1).

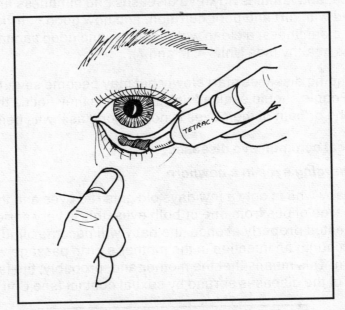

If the mother and baby cannot go to the hospital or to the health centre, ask your supervisor to come to see the baby.

In the meantime, wash the baby's eyes as described above, and keep the eyes clear of discharge. Put tetracycline eye ointment under the eyelids 5 times a day until the discharge has stopped. Then continue with the ointment 3 times a day for 3 more days.

Give the baby the same injection of procaine benzylpenicillin twice a day for 3 days (a total of 6 injections). Examine the baby daily for 3 more days.

If you have no eye ointment or penicillin injection, send *at once* for your supervisor or for a nurse or doctor from the health centre.

> **Note**
>
> *In some places penicillin should not be used for this disease. When you study this problem, you should ask your supervisor or the doctor in the health centre what is the recommended treatment in your country.*

The mother and father of this child also need treatment. If they can go to the health centre or hospital, they will get the treatment there. If they cannot go to the hospital or health centre, treat as described in Unit 43 "Venereal diseases" page 320.

Prevention. To prevent this disease of newborn babies, see Units 16 and 17, pages 127 and 146.

A red discharging eye in a child or adult

A person with a red eye and a discharge of pus should:

- Wash the face with soap and water and the eyes with water 3 times a day.

- Put tetracycline eye ointment into *both* eyes 3 times a day for 5 days (see Annex 1).

- Keep the hands clean by washing them with soap and water several times a day.

If after 5 days there is no more discharge, the patient is cured. Otherwise send the patient to the health centre or hospital.

A red, cloudy eye

When the eye is red and the clear front part of the eye (the cornea) has an area or spot that is no longer clear, treat the person as follows:

Clean the eye with a freshly washed, damp cloth, put tetracycline eye ointment under the eyelids, and send the patient at once to the health centre or hospital.

A red, painful eye

When a person has a red eye that is painful and has lost some sight, send him at once to the health centre or hospital.

Eye diseases that come gradually

Any person who has lost sight in one or both eyes, even if there is no pain, should be sent to the health centre or hospital.

If, in a child, the surface of the eye appears dry, or the child does not see well in the evening, it usually means that the child lacks vitamin A. If you can, give the child a capsule of retinol (see Annex 1) by mouth once. If you have no retinol, send the child to the health centre at once, or ask for your supervisor's help.

Explain to the parents that the child will become blind unless he regularly eats food that contains vitamin A: carrots, fruits such as papaya and mangoes, and green leafy vegetables. The schoolteacher should know this and remind the pupils of it from time to time.

Children also often get an eye infection called **trachoma**. It makes the inside of the eyelids rough and red. The treatment is to put tetracycline eye ointment on the inside of the eyelids every day for 6 weeks. The child's face and eyes should be washed carefully every day.

Loss of sight in old people

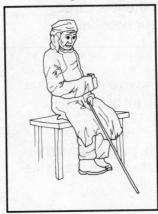

This is usually a clouding of the eye (**a cataract**). After some time, light cannot pass through the eye and the old person becomes completely blind. Eye-drops, pills and injections do not help, but the sight can come back again after a surgical operation. Therefore, you should write down the patient's name and address so that you can let the family know when and where the next eye camp will be, or you should send the patient to a health centre or hospital.

How to treat common injuries of the eye

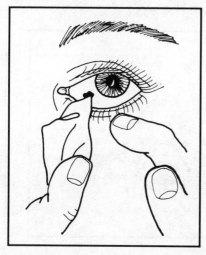

(1) When a piece of dirt, sand, or other particle gets into the eye or underneath an eyelid it may injure the eye. Try to remove it by wiping gently the surface of the eye or the inside of the eyelid with a clean cloth (see drawing), or try to wash it out by bathing the eye with clean water in a small clean cup or tablespoon.

Put tetracycline eye ointment under the eyelid, and ask the patient to come to see you if the eye is painful again.

If you cannot remove the particle or if the eye continues to hurt, send the patient to the health centre or hospital.

(2) When there is a scratch on the surface of the eye put tetracycline eye ointment under the eyelids 3 times a day for 3 days and cover the eye with a pad and a light bandage. If there is no improvement in 3 days, refer the patient to the health centre or hospital.

(3) When the eyelid is torn or there is a wound of the eyeball, put a clean dressing on it, and send the patient to hospital at once. ***Do not put any drops or ointment on or into the eye.*** If the patient cannot get to a hospital or health centre within 2–3 hours, give tetracycline by mouth or penicillin by injection (see Annex 1).

How to fold the eyelid back and remove something from the eye:

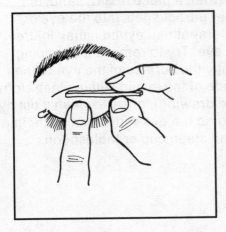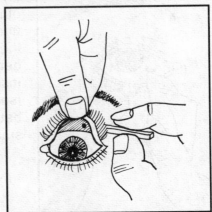

Hold the edge of the eyelid between the thumb and the index finger. Gently pull it down a little. Fold the eyelid back over a matchstick held in the other hand. Remove the particle with a clean cloth as described above. Put a little tetracycline eye ointment (as much as a drop of water) on to the eyelid (see Annex 1).

(4) When there is a burn of the eye, whether by fire, heat, or chemicals, do the following:

- wash the burned eye at once with a lot of clean water

- put tetracycline eye ointment under the eyelids

- send the patient at once to the health centre or hospital.

Test for sight

The person should cover one eye with his hand. You stand 6 metres away from him, and hold up any number of fingers on one of your hands. Ask the person to tell you or show you how many fingers you are holding up.

If he cannot see your fingers properly, the sight in that eye is seriously damaged. Repeat this with the other eye.

If he cannot count your fingers from 6 metres with either eye, send him to the health centre or hospital.

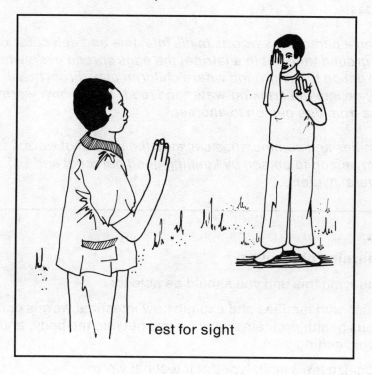

Test for sight

293

Intestinal worms

Intestinal worms may be found in the soil, water, and food in all countries. They get into the body with contaminated food or through the skin. Then they live in the patient's intestine. They live on the food that the patient eats, and this makes the patient's body weak and tired.

The worms lay eggs inside the body, which come out in the faeces.

When a person has worms in his intestine and defecates on the ground (and not in a latrine) the eggs spread everywhere and get on to the ground where children play. From there they go into the drinking-water and food. This is how worms pass from one person to another.

Families and communities can stop the spread of worms from person to person by keeping good personal and general hygiene.

Learning objectives

After studying this unit you should be able to:

1 Discuss with families and explain how intestinal worms cause serious health problems, how worms get into the body, and how to avoid getting them.

2 Recognize the 3 main types of intestinal worm.

3 Treat a patient and the household of a patient who is passing roundworms, tapeworms, or pinworms (threadworms).

4 Advise that:

- all members of a family or community should be treated and not just the person you know has worms

- any child who has worms and severe pains in the belly should be sent to the health centre or hospital.

Discuss the problem of intestinal worms with the community

You should discuss the problem of intestinal worms with community groups, the community committee, the women's group, schoolteachers, and schoolchildren.

First find out how common the problem of intestinal worms is in your community. Tell your supervisor about it if it deserves special attention.

Remind people that they get intestinal worms because:

- they eat without washing hands after passing faeces or after working or playing on the ground with mud, etc.
- they eat vegetables and fruit contaminated with soil in which there are eggs of intestinal worms without washing them first
- they eat beef or pork that has worms and which is raw or not very well cooked
- they drink dirty water
- they go barefoot on ground contaminated with faeces.

Tell the people that they can protect themselves against intestinal worms by:

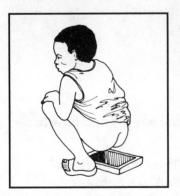 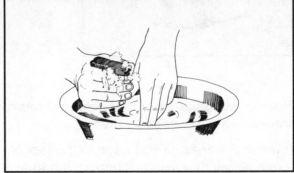

- defecating in a latrine and keeping the latrine clean (see Unit 7)
- washing hands with soap and water after defecating and after working or playing on the ground and before eating food

295

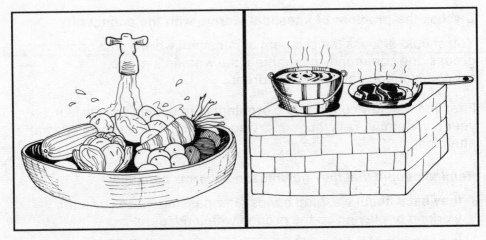

- washing fruit and vegetables well with clean water
- eating only well-cooked meat

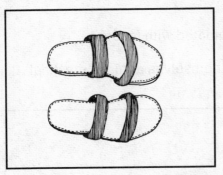

- wearing shoes or sandals
- drinking clean water (see Unit 4).

How to recognize the 3 main types of intestinal worms and how to treat diseases caused by them

Intestinal worms can be seen in the faeces. They may be round like a pencil, flat like a ribbon, or small and thin like a thread.

The worm is round and long like a pencil

The mother has seen roundworms in the child's faeces. The child has no complaints, but sometimes has a little pain in the belly.

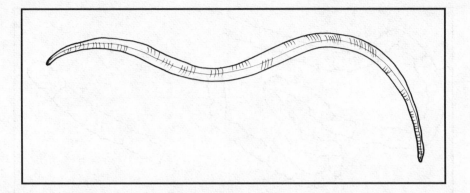

Give this child mebendazole or piperazine tablets (see Annex 1). Ask the parents whether others in the family or community have worms, and, if so, treat them at the same time.

If a child or an adult has worms and bad pains in the belly, send the patient to the hospital or health centre.

Important!

Tell the family that they will get worms again unless they:

- *use a clean latrine*
- *wash their hands well before they eat and after they defecate*
- *drink only safe water*
- *do not eat food contaminated with soil until it has been well washed with clean water.*

The worm is flat like a ribbon and has segments (rings)

This is a tapeworm. Parts of it (several segments or rings) can be seen in the faeces. Some rings may also appear in the underwear. A person who has a tapeworm may have pains in the belly.

Give the patient niclosamide tablets (see Annex 1). Ask whether

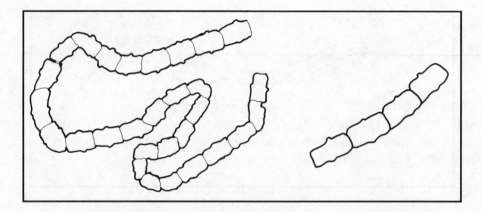

others in the family have seen tapeworms in their faeces and, if so, *treat them* as well.

Repeat the advice on cleanliness. Insist that beef and pork must always be well cooked.

The worms are short and thin like a thread

These worms are called pinworms or threadworms. If a child has these worms, the skin around his anus will itch after he goes to bed. If you examine this child you will be able to see the worms on the skin around the anus. When you examine the child make sure there is enough light in the room (or use a torch).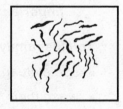

Give the patient mebendazole or piperazine tablets (see Annex 1).

Usually when one child in a house has pinworms, all the children, and often the adults too, will have them. It is of no use then to treat only one person. All should be treated at the same time.

Other worms

There are also other kinds of intestinal worms such as hookworms, which are also short and thin, but they cannot be seen easily in the faeces. They cause anaemia (see Unit 39) and weakness and tiredness. A patient with anaemia is likely to have hookworms if hookworm infection is common in your area and if there are no other reasons for the anaemia (such as malnutrition or malaria). Give the patient mebendazole and iron sulfate tablets (see Annex 1).

The patient and the family should defecate in a latrine and wear shoes or sandals especially when walking or squatting on ground where people defecate. The hookworm enters the body through the soles of the feet, and shoes or sandals can prevent this happening.

If there is no improvement in the weakness and tiredness after 4 weeks, send the patient to the health centre or hospital.

Remember!

When someone has intestinal worms, you should see whether others in the family or in the community also have worms. All those who are infected should be treated at the same time; if you do not do this, those who are not treated will quickly pass on the worms to those who have been treated.

It is good to treat people who have worms, but it is even better to prevent people from getting them. The people themselves can do the most to get rid of intestinal worms from the community by improving sanitation in their village and at home, and practising cleanliness as indicated above.

Weakness and tiredness

Many patients complain of feeling weak and tired. There are many causes for this. A common cause is hunger when food is scarce or families have too little money to buy good food.

Weakness and tiredness can be signs of several serious diseases. In some of those diseases patients lose blood, and even a small loss of blood can make a patient weak and tired. Weakness and tiredness can also be a sign of a mental disorder.

Learning objectives

After studying this unit you should be able to:

1 Find out what makes a person feel weak and tired.

2 Decide when a person who complains of weakness and tiredness should go to the health centre or hospital.

3 Treat and advise a person who is weak and tired and has not been sent to the health centre or hospital.

4 Discuss with a family what they should eat to keep everybody strong and in good health.

5 Discuss with the community committee what can be done to increase the availability and use of foods so that people can keep strong and healthy.

How long has the patient been feeling weak and tired?

If a patient complains of weakness and tiredness, find out how long he or she has been feeling that way.

The patient has felt weak and tired suddenly

If the patient suddenly felt weak and collapsed (fell down), ask the patient or the people around what happened:

- Did the person have an accident (and if yes, of what kind)?
- Has he lost a lot of blood?
- Has he belly pains?
- Is he unconscious?

If yes, send him to the hospital immediately.

The patient has felt weak and tired for some time

(1) *Weakness and tiredness plus other problems*

Weakness and tiredness are common signs of many diseases. Check whether there is also: fever, cough, diarrhoea, headaches, bleeding, belly pains, poisoning, pains in the joints in children or young people, intestinal worms, blood in the urine. If any of these problems is present, treat according to the instructions given in corresponding units in this book.

Also find out:

- Has the patient lost weight recently?
- Has he lost his appetite?
- Has he difficulty in breathing?
- Has he had pain in the chest?
- Does he sweat heavily in bed at night?
- Is the skin, the inside of the eyelids or the white part of the eye, or the urine yellow?
- Are the ankles swollen?

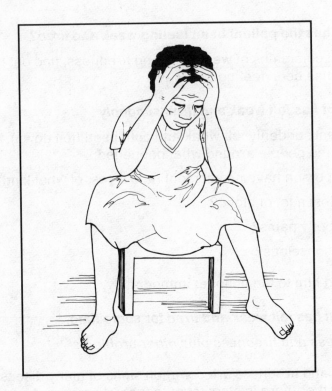

If the answer to one or more of these questions is "yes", send the patient to the health centre or hospital without delay.

If the answer to all the above questions is "no", find out:

- Does the patient wake from sleep very early and feel sad all the time?

- Does the patient have many different complaints such as headache, loss of appetite, sexual difficulties, hot feelings or a feeling of tightness in the head?

If the answer to one or both of these questions is yes, treat according to instructions given in Unit 42 "Mental health and mental disorders".

(2) *Weakness and tiredness in children*

If the patient is a child, who appears weak and tired all the time, check his growth chart to see whether the child is gaining weight normally and whether the child is feeding properly (see Unit 20).

(3) Weakness and tiredness in women

First see if the woman has any other complaint such as fever, cough, etc.; then check if she has any mental problems (see (1) above). If she has none of these, look for the following signs and treat according to the instructions given in the appropriate units (Units 15 and 19):

- pregnancy or recent childbirth
- heavy periods
- other bleeding from the vagina
- frequent pregnancies (short interval between pregnancies).

If the inside of the woman's eyelids is pale (it should normally be red or pink), the woman has anaemia (or thin blood). This is caused either by blood loss or lack of iron in the diet. Give her iron sulfate tablets (see Annex 1). Also advise her to eat foods that are rich in iron every day. The best such foods are liver, red meat, chicken, fish and eggs, as well as dark green leafy vegetables and pulses (peas, beans, lentils).

If she does not begin to feel strong in 3–4 weeks, or if she becomes worse, send her to the health centre.

If she feels better in that time, continue to give her iron sulfate tablets.

If the woman cannot have some of these foods every day or at least 3 times a week, because they are hard to find or the family has not enough money to buy them, she will continue to feel weak and tired and she may not be able to care well for her children. You should tell the community committee about this problem and discuss with a women's group in the community how this woman can be helped.

Keeping the mouth and teeth healthy

People need healthy teeth and gums to be able to eat well, speak well, and have pleasant breath, a good appearance, and good general health.

If people eat too much sweet food and drink too many sweet drinks, their teeth will decay and their gums will become unhealthy. If people always clean their teeth after meals, they will prevent little bits of food from staying between the teeth and damaging them. This damage can begin in childhood and parents may not notice it until a lot of damage has been done. There will then be much pain and the teeth will fall out.

Learning objectives

After studying this unit you should be able to:

1 Explain to people why the mouth and teeth should be kept healthy, and how to do so.

2 Suspect tetanus in a patient who cannot open the mouth and send him to the hospital or health centre at once.

3 Give first aid to, and advise, a patient whose mouth or teeth hurt, and refer to the health centre all serious cases for special dental care.

Three good habits to suggest

You should explain to those coming to see you with teeth problems, and to various groups in your community, especially schoolchildren and women, how to keep the mouth and teeth healthy.

Clean the mouth and teeth after meals

After each meal we should all clean our teeth, clean between them and rinse the mouth with water. Cleaning of teeth should be done with a chewing stick, or when possible, a toothbrush and toothpaste containing fluoride.

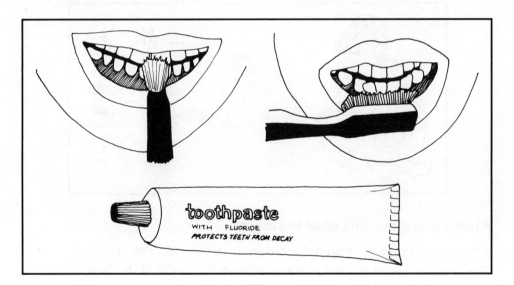

Do not give children too many sweets

Children should not eat too many sweets, sugar, cakes, or sweet drinks, especially between meals.

Eat and drink food that protects the health of the teeth

Such foods are: breast milk (for babies), cow's or buffalo's milk (for children), fresh fruit and vegetables, coconut, taro, sweet potato, etc.

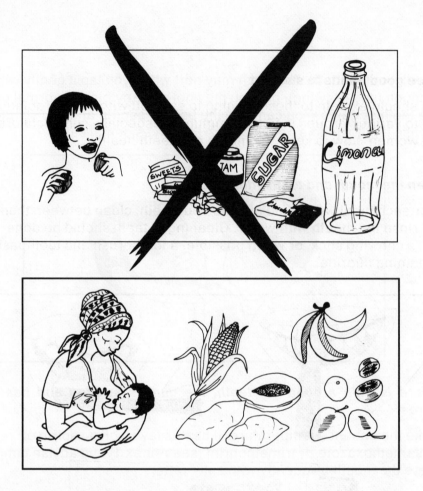

When a patient cannot open the mouth

If the patient has not had an accident or a blow on the jaw, but has had a cut or a wound somewhere on the body in the last 10 days or so, you should suspect tetanus (lockjaw). This is a very serious disease. The patient will die if he is not treated immediately. Send the patient to the hospital or health centre at once.

Most often when the mouth or teeth hurt the patient can open the mouth

Toothache (pain in a tooth)

If a person has pain in a tooth, especially when eating or drinking something hot or cold, this usually means that there is a hole (cavity) in the tooth. The tooth may hurt when you tap it gently with a spoon (see drawing), but you may not see anything abnormal on the tooth or gums. You can give the patient aspirin and you should advise him to go to a health centre that gives dental care.

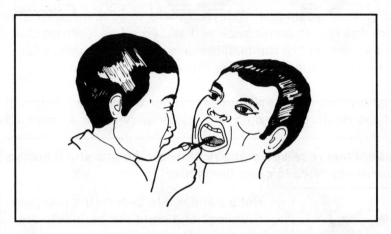

There is pain around the teeth, the gum is swollen and has little sores

Take the patient's temperature. If he has fever, give aspirin or sulfamethoxazole + trimethoprim (see Annex 1) and advise him to rinse the mouth frequently with salty water.

See the patient again after 3 days and tap each tooth with a spoon. If no tooth hurts, advise the patient about the care of the mouth and teeth as above (see page 305). If a tooth hurts, advise the patient to go for treatment, if possible to a health centre that gives dental care.

If the patient has no fever, advise a mouthwash 4 times a day for 1 week (see drawings on pages 308–309).

Something hurts in the mouth

If there is a swelling or small sores in the mouth, but not around the teeth, send the patient to the health centre or hospital.

Something hurts only when the patient swallows (sore throat)

Take the patient's temperature. If the patient has fever, give aspirin or sulfamethoxazole + trimethoprim (see Annex 1).

See the patient again after 3 days. If there is no fever, the patient is cured. Ask him to come back and see you if he feels tired or if he has swollen feet or joints. If there is no improvement after 3 days, send the patient to the health centre or hospital.

If the patient has no fever, give aspirin for 3 days (see Annex 1) and advise rinsing the mouth with warm salty water 4 times a day.

The patient has received a heavy blow on the jaw and it hurts a lot when he or she tries to open the mouth

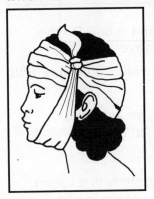

Put a bandage to secure the jaw (see drawing) and send the patient to the hospital or health centre.

Mouthwash

1 Fill the mouth with salty water.

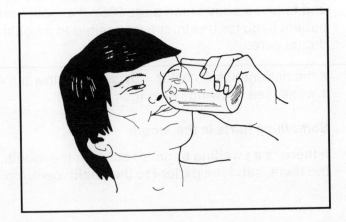

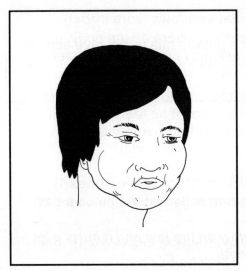

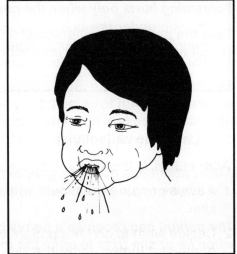

2 Do not swallow it but move it around the mouth 5 or 6 times.

3 Then spit it out. Do this again several times.

Lumps under the skin

A lump under the skin can appear anywhere on the body. It may be a swollen gland, especially if it is in the neck, under the arm, or in the groin. It may also be in a breast.

Learning objectives

After studying this unit you should be able to:

1 Advise people how to reduce the risk of getting lumps under the skin.

2 Decide what to do for a patient who comes to see you with one or several lumps under the skin, which he has had

- for only a few days, or

- for more than 2 weeks.

3 Show a patient how to make and use a hot compress.

What do lumps under the skin indicate?

(1) If the lump is hard and painful and the skin over it is red and hot, it means there is an infection under the skin (perhaps with pus). Such a lump is called a **boil** or **abscess**.

(2) If there is a lump in the neck, armpit, or groin, it means that there is an infection in the neck or head, in the arm or hand, or in the leg or foot, respectively. Such lumps occur when glands in the neck, armpit, or groin swell up because of the infection.

(3) If a woman has lumps in the breasts, it may mean there is a serious disease. She should go to the health centre as soon as possible (see also Unit 19).

How to reduce the risk of getting lumps under the skin

Lumps may appear under the skin if people:

- do not wash the whole body regularly with soap and water to get rid of dust and sweat
- do not wash their clothes regularly
- are not properly treated for a wound or a skin disease
- do not eat well and are tired
- have been bitten by a fly or other insect.

To reduce this problem in the community advise the people:

- to keep their bodies clean
- to wear clean clothes
- to come and see you about any wound, any skin disease or any bad insect bite
- to eat well and sleep sufficiently.

A patient has one or more lumps under the skin

First, ask how long the lump has been there.

The lump has been there for only a few days

Take the patient's temperature. If the patient is feverish, the lump hurts, and the skin over the lump is red and hot, show the patient how to put hot compresses on the lump (see drawing) and give the patient aspirin.

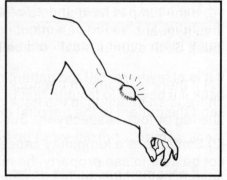

See the patient again the next day. If the fever has gone, tell him to keep the skin clean until the lump goes away.

If the lump has opened and there is pus coming out, treat it as a wound (see Unit 31).

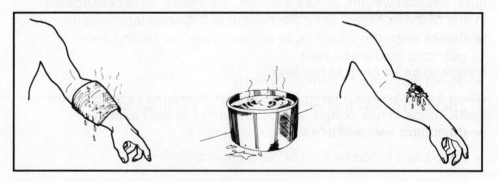

If the patient is still feverish and the lump hurts a lot send him to the hospital or health centre.

If the patient is feverish and the lump does not hurt, tell the patient to wash the skin over the lump and give him aspirin.

See the patient again next day. If there is still fever, send him to the hospital or health centre.

The lump has been there for more than 2 weeks

(1) The lump has been there for some time, and it does not trouble the patient in his life or work. If it is in a breast, see "A woman has a lump in her breast" below (also see Unit 19).

If it is elsewhere, tell the patient not to worry about it, but to come back if it begins to trouble him in his life or his work. In that case, send the patient to the hospital or health centre.

(2) Sometimes a lump may cause the patient some trouble. He may not be able to see properly, he may not be able to hear properly, he may have difficulty in swallowing or breathing, he may be constipated, or he may not be able to work or walk. Send the patient to the hospital or health centre.

Sometimes a patient who has a lump in his body feels tired, eats little, has lost weight, or has a cough, diarrhoea, or is constipated. In any of these cases, send the patient to the hospital or health centre.

A woman has a lump in her breast

When a woman has a lump in her breast, there may also be a few small lumps in her armpit (axilla). Send her to the hospital or health centre without delay (see also Unit 19).

Remember!

The most dangerous lumps are those you can feel:

- *around the neck (in front, at the side, or back)*
- *in the armpit*
- *in the groin*
- *in the breast.*

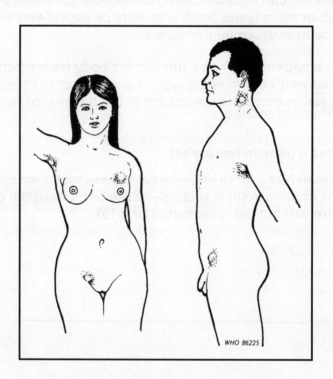

WHO 86225

Unit 42
Mental health and mental disorders

To be in good health is to be healthy in body and mind. People are mentally healthy when they are happy to be alive and like living with other people. They try to solve their own problems, receive help when needed, and can help other people to solve their problems.

Mental disorders are those that affect people's minds, feelings, and behaviour.

Healers or religious leaders often treat and advise people who have mental disorders. You should keep in touch with these healers and offer them your help or ask for their help when you need it.

Learning objectives

After studying this unit you should be able to:

1 Identify patients with a mental disorder.

2 Encourage patients to try to solve their own problems with the help of their relatives, friends, or other people in the community.

3 Tell which persons with mental disorder should go to the health centre or hospital.

Patients with mental disorders

Patients who behave in a strange way

You will easily recognize these people, or their families or neighbours will tell you about them, because they do not behave as others do. They may:

- be violent, angry, or may shout or fight without any reason

- behave in a way that people do not like

- look lost and not know where they are

- be too quiet and not want to talk to anybody

- hear voices and see things that other people do not hear or see

- no longer wash, dress or work

- be very sad and cry without any reason

- threaten to kill themselves

- have lost their memory

- run away from home

- drink too much alcohol or take drugs

- have difficulty, or be very slow, in learning.

Patients with vague complaints

You will recognize these patients because they have many complaints of many kinds which are not specific diseases. They may tell you, for instance, that:

- they feel weak and get tired easily

- they have pains or strange feelings in their head, their belly, their arms, their legs

■ they have no appetite

■ they have a hot feeling in their head, or a tight feeling, or it feels as if something heavy is pressing down on their head

■ they have difficulty in getting to sleep, or they keep waking up for no reason

■ they have difficulties in their sexual life.

What can you do?

If the patient is not violent and the problem is not new

A mental health problem is not urgent if it has lasted for some time already, and the patient is not violent. In such a case, do not give any drug but talk with the family, seek the advice of the local community or religious leaders or healers, and try to provide useful ideas and common sense to help the patient and his family to solve their problems.

Talk also with your supervisor who may suggest that the patient be taken to the hospital or health centre.

If the patient is violent

A mental health problem becomes serious and needs immediate action when you think there may be a danger to the patient or to other people. The following need immediate help:

(1) *A person who has drunk too much alcohol and has become violent*

First, you should arrange for the person to sleep, and then, you should meet him with his family and explain that alcohol harms health in several ways. It can:

■ damage the liver and the brain

■ cause loss of sexual power

■ make the body unable to fight against infections

317

■ cause a person to become addicted (that is, unable to stop drinking alcohol)

■ cause a person to become violent or useless and to lose everything he owns.

Discuss with the family how the person can be helped to drink less or to give up drinking altogether. If he still keeps on drinking too much, advise the family to take him to the health centre or hospital.

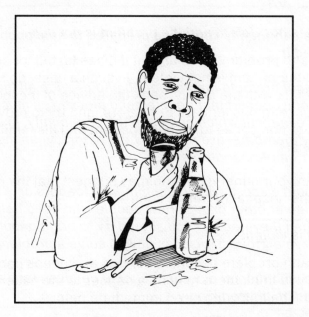

(2) *A person who has taken drugs* (e.g., hashish, cannabis, opium, heroin)

Drugs can have the same harmful effects as alcohol. Discuss with the family and the community to decide what can be done.

(3) *A person who is very excited*

Ask the people around him to leave you alone with him. Try to calm him by talking to him. Give him some water to drink. Check whether he has fever (fever sometimes causes abnormal or strange behaviour).

If you do not succeed in calming him or if he becomes excited again, advise the family to take him to the health centre or hospital.

(4) *A person who talks of killing himself*

Listen to him and discuss his problem with him. Ask someone to stay with him. Advise the family to take him to the health centre or hospital.

The community should be prepared to help people who need it

You cannot promote mental health and provide all the social and mental support that people need alone. You must therefore find out which people in the community, in addition to family members, are ready to help others when they have social or emotional problems.

You should discuss with the community leaders or committee or other groups how people who need help can get it when they need it. You should try to bring people together in a group to discuss how to solve a problem.

Patients with mental disorders should be given food and drink and be treated kindly.

Venereal diseases

These are the diseases that an infected man or woman may pass on to his or her partner during sexual intercourse. For this reason they are called sexually transmitted diseases. They are also called venereal diseases.

In many places they affect a large number of young people.

You should always treat all partners at the same time, if possible.

In order to be able to discuss diseases of the sexual organs patients must have confidence in you. This means they believe that you know how to treat them, that you will not tell anyone about their problems, and that you will make it easy for them to discuss them with you.

Learning objectives

After studying this unit you should be able to:

1 Treat a man who has a white or yellow discharge from his penis.

2 Treat a woman who has a white or yellow discharge from her vagina.

3 Recognize a sore (ulcer) on the genitals and treat a man or a woman with such a sore.

4 Treat a man or a woman with lumps (enlarged glands) in the groin.

5 Discuss with the community leaders and groups how these diseases are spread, what their effects may be, and how to prevent them.

A man with a discharge from the penis (drawing 2)

The discharge is white or yellow (whitish yellow) and usually there is pain while urinating.

Give the patient tetracycline tablets: 2 tablets (250 mg each) 4 times a day for 7 days (a total of 56 tablets). Ask the patient to take them between meals (see Annex 1).

If there is no discharge at the end of this treatment, the patient is cured.

If there is still discharge, send the patient to the health centre or hospital.

All his sexual partners during the past two weeks should be given the same treatment.

A woman with a discharge from the vagina (drawing 1)

With the discharge there may or may not be pain in the lower part of the belly.

Give the patient tetracycline tablets: 2 tablets (250 mg each) 4 times a day for 7 days (a total of 56 tablets). The tablets should be taken between meals (see Annex 1).

If the discharge has not gone away at the end of this treatment give the patient 2 g of metronidazole by mouth (one dose). If you have 500-mg tablets give 4 of them to be taken at once (see Annex 1).

If the discharge has not gone away after 2 days, send the patient to the health centre or hospital.

All sexual partners of the woman during the past month should be given the same treatment.

A woman with a severe pain in the lower part of the belly after a vaginal discharge should be sent to the hospital as soon as possible. If this is not possible, give her tetracycline as above.

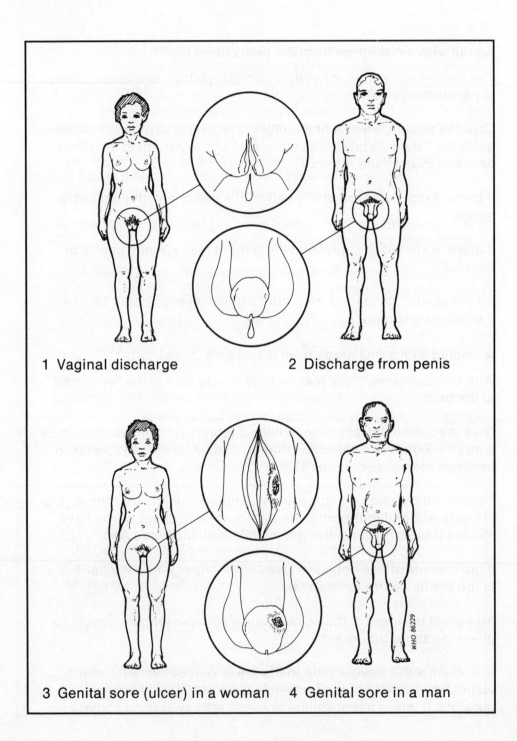

1 Vaginal discharge   2 Discharge from penis

3 Genital sore (ulcer) in a woman   4 Genital sore in a man

WHO 86229

A man or a woman has a small sore (ulcer) on the genitals, sometimes with lumps in the groin (drawings 3 and 4)

Give the patient one injection of benzathine benzylpenicillin (2.4 million units) into the buttock. (If you have no benzathine benzylpenicillin, send the patient to the health centre or hospital.)

If the sore is not healed after 4 days, give a supply of tablets of sulfamethoxazole + trimethoprim. The patient should take 8 tablets each day for 2 days (4 tablets in the morning, 4 in the evening).

If the sore does not start to heal in 4 days after this treatment, send the patient to the health centre or hospital.

All the patient's sexual partners during the past month should be given the same treatment.

A man or a woman has lumps in the groin (large lymph nodes)

If there is also a sore (ulcer) on the genitals give the same treatment as that for a genital sore (see above).

If there is no sore or it has healed, give the patient tetracycline, 2 tablets 4 times a day for 7 days (a total of 56 tablets).

If the lumps do not become much smaller after this treatment, send the patient to the health centre or hospital.

Remember!

- *People with a venereal disease pass on the infection to their partner during sexual intercourse. Often, people who have these diseases do not know that they have them, or they pay no attention to them.*

- *Sexual intercourse with more than one partner increases the risk of catching these diseases.*

- *If the genitals are not washed daily, and especially after each intercourse, the risk of venereal diseases increases.*

How to prevent venereal diseases

Tell the people in your community that to avoid these diseases they should:

- avoid sexual intercourse with people who have many partners

- keep very clean by always washing their genitals with soap and water, especially after sexual intercourse

- ensure that sexual partners of patients with venereal diseases are treated, so that these diseases cannot be passed to others

- use condoms (see Unit 18).

A man or woman who thinks that he or she has a venereal disease, should go for examination and treatment as soon as possible. Venereal diseases are easy to treat at the beginning, but more difficult to treat later.

What can happen if these diseases are not properly treated at once?

(1) If the infection is not treated, it will pass from the outer to the inner sexual organs: the womb, the tubes, the ovaries (in women) and the testes (in man). This can cause severe acute illness at first, and, later, the woman may become sterile (unable to become pregnant), or may have repeated miscarriages or stillbirths (babies born dead). The man may also become sterile (unable to make babies).

(2) The disease will spread to other sexual partners of the infected persons.

(3) Babies may be born with a venereal disease if the mother has a venereal disease that has not been treated (see Unit 37).

Unit 44

Blood in the urine

Children and others who have blood in their urine may have a disease called schistosomiasis (or bilharziasis). Find out the name used in your community and use that name when you talk about this disease.

You have seen in Unit 9 "Vectors of disease" that snails in water or on damp ground can carry a worm which causes schistosomiasis. The disease is caused when the worm enters the body through the skin when people are washing or swimming in a river or an irrigation canal.

Schistosomiasis does not occur everywhere. It occurs in tropical areas where there are snails, water, and vegetation. In some places many or most of the children pass blood in their urine. This means that the worm that causes schistosomiasis is living in their bodies (urinary bladders).

Learning objectives

After studying this unit you should be able to:

1 Find the schoolchildren in your area who have schistosomiasis.

2 Discuss with families and the community how to stop the disease.

3 Arrange for all who have the disease to receive treatment.

4 Cooperate with the health service in action against the disease.

Schistosomiasis weakens children, prevents them from growing properly, and makes them less resistant to infections.

First, with the help of the teachers, ask the schoolchildren:

- whether they have blood in their urine, or
- whether they have had blood in the urine within the past month.

Treatment can stop the disease from spreading

Explain to the community, and especially to the schoolchildren, that this disease can be stopped if all the people who have blood in the urine take treatment from the health centre at about the same time. This means that adults with blood in their urine should be treated at the same time as children. Explain also why people should:

- not urinate in or near water
- use latrines properly
- not swim or bathe or wash clothes in water where there are snails.

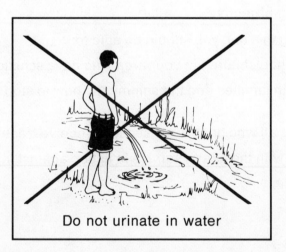

Do not urinate in water

Arrange for all those who have the disease to go to the health centre to be treated *or* arrange for someone from the health centre to come to your village to treat all the patients at the same time.

How you can help in preventing the disease

Discuss with your supervisor what you can do to cooperate in any action taken against schistosomiasis, for example:

- Help in clearing all vegetation from the water where people swim or bathe or wash clothes.

- Cooperate with the health service in diagnosing and treating all the people who are infected in your village.

- Follow up once a year for two or three years children who have received treatment to check whether they have stopped having blood in their urine. If they still have blood in the urine, inform your supervisor.

See also Units 4, 7, 8, and 9.

Epilepsy (fits)

Some people have a weakness in the brain that causes them to fall down unconscious in a fit (convulsion) and to shake, often foaming at the mouth and sometimes urinating. This is epilepsy. Every language has a word for this disease (e.g., falling sickness). The fits can occur once or more every month or less often. Sometimes a person may have several fits within a few days and then none for several weeks or months.

These fits can be prevented or very much reduced by medicines and the patients can lead normal lives like other people.

When a young child with a high fever has a fit this is usually not epilepsy.

Learning objectives

After studying this unit you should be able to:

1 Recognize an epileptic fit.

2 Show people what to do when someone is having a fit.

3 Prevent fits by convincing the patient to take continuous drug treatment.

4 Discuss with the community the social problems that come with epilepsy.

What to do during a fit

Advise the patient's family members about what to do if the patient has a fit. Tell them to:

- keep calm and not be afraid
- let the patient lie down in a safe place out of the way of traffic or a fire
- fold a cloth and put it under the patient's head, or hold the head so that it does not bang on hard things
- loosen any tight clothing
- turn the patient to lie on one side so that the tongue comes to the front of the mouth and froth can come out of the mouth easily
- stay with the patient until the fit is over and he is awake again.

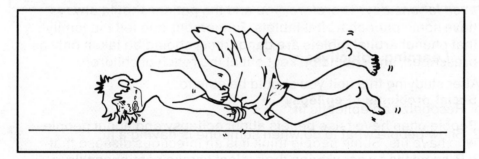

During the fit:

- try to prevent the patient from biting his tongue
- do not give anything to eat or drink
- do not give any herbs or medicine
- do not try to stop or control the shaking movements.

After the fit, the patient goes into a deep sleep. Keep him on his side and let him rest.

How to prevent fits by continuous treatment

When a person has had fits several times without having fever, it is probably epilepsy. If possible, send the patient to a health centre or hospital. If this is not possible at once, begin treatment to prevent more fits, but make sure the patient goes to the health centre as soon as possible.

Give phenobarbital (see Annex 1).

Find out from the health centre what the continuous treatment is and make sure you have a supply of the drug. Make sure the parents or relatives understand that a child (or adult) with epilepsy should take the treatment all the time and should be seen regularly at the health centre. Usually the fits will not happen if the patient takes phenobarbital tablets every day. The tablets will need to be given for several years and should *never* be stopped suddenly, *not even for one day*. Therefore, you and the patient should always have some phenobarbital tablets. Remember and tell the family that phenobarbital tablets are dangerous, should be taken only as prescribed, and should be kept out of the reach of children.

Social problems of epilepsy

People often have false beliefs about epilepsy and about people who have fits. Some people think it is an infectious disease that can be passed on to others, or that it is shameful to have this disease and that the epileptic patient should not mix with other people. As part of the care of the patient, he should be protected from those false beliefs. You should discuss with the people what they believe and what you have learned about epilepsy.

The family of the patient and the community should know that:

- Epilepsy is caused by a very small weakness in the brain.

- Most patients can live normal lives in spite of the fits. Children who get fits can go to school and learn normally. They should be accepted as normal people.

- Patients can have tablets to prevent the fits.

- Epilepsy is not infectious. It cannot be passed from one person to another.

- The froth that comes from the mouth in a fit is not harmful.

Other kinds of fits

Some children under 6 years old may have a convulsion during a high fever. If this happens only once or twice it is not epilepsy.

Chapter 7
Getting the work done

Unit 46
Home visiting

Home visits are an important part of your work. Many times the only way you can get information you need is to visit a family at home. Sometimes the only way you can teach someone in a family how to give better care to a sick or disabled member is to show them how to do so in their home using the family's own things.

Learning objectives

After studying this unit you should be able to:

1 Explain to community leaders and families the main rules of home visiting.

2 Give them 3 reasons for making a home visit.

3 Plan your home-visiting day and take only what you need to make your visits successful.

4 Record what you have done, what you have seen, and what was decided.

The main rules of home visiting

When making a home visit, remember:

(1) You are a visitor. Therefore, obey the customary rules for visiting any house even if you know the household very well. Never go inside until you have been invited.

(2) You are there to help the family to identify or solve its health problems or to check up on health action they have promised to take. They may have a lot of work to do: you should not waste their time with unnecessary talk.

(3) Many households you will visit may have very little of their basic needs (water, food, soap, etc.). Use them carefully. If they invite you to eat with them, for example, make sure first that

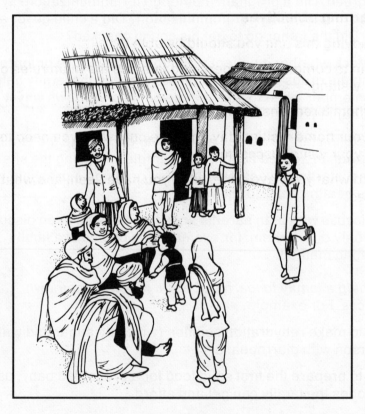

everyone has enough to eat. If you think that they do not have enough food, make some excuse or only accept a small drink.

(4) Do not be too critical, or they may not allow you to visit again. Be positive. For example: "You seem to have a lot of flies in the house. Would you like us to find out together where they come from? Flies carry a lot of sickness. Getting rid of them would make you healthier."

Main reasons for making home visits

(1) *To help a family become healthier or to find out how the family is following the advice given previously.* Some examples of reasons for home visiting are:

- To find out whether the family members went to the health post as agreed. Did a pregnant mother go for immunization? Was a newborn baby taken for immunization? Did a child go for an eye test? Did the father go to get his cough checked?

- To check whether a patient with tuberculosis (TB) or leprosy is taking the drugs given, and that someone in the family helps him to remember when to take the medicine and knows why it is important to do so.

- To help to start an agreed action or to encourage the family to carry out an agreed action, for example, choosing the site for a latrine, starting a vegetable garden, or taking a pregnant woman to the health centre for delivery.

- To discuss with both parents an action that has been discussed with only one of them, for example, the choice of a family planning method.

(2) *To help a family to learn a specific skill with their own resources.* For example:

- how to make rehydration solution (with salt, sugar and water) for a person with diarrhoea, or

- how to prepare the first solid food for a breast-fed baby, using the foods the family can get and afford.

(3) *To collect information.* For example:

- To carry out a survey to find out who lives in each house in the village (see Unit 1).

- To find out how each family lives and whether the place where they live is itself a cause of their health problems (see Unit 3).

- To find out how the different family members behave and who influences what the family does. You should give this person new ideas for family health to make sure the family accepts them and puts them into action.

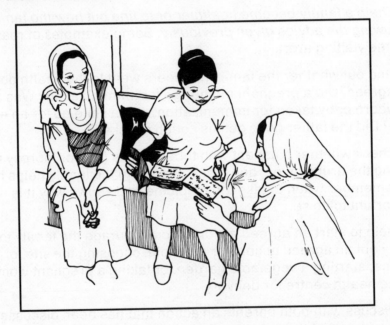

Planning home visits

Deciding whom to visit

You may have a very long list of households that you feel you should visit. You cannot visit all of them. Try to divide the visits on your list into "very important" and "least important", or into tasks "to do at once" and those "to do if I am in the area". Ask your supervisor to help you set these priorities for your community.

Take advantage of other services

For example, if the immunization team is coming to your area and you are going to help, visit at the same time the families who have a health problem but whom you cannot visit often.

If the agriculture truck is going to a distant place, go in it to visit families who also live in that area. At the same time, visit the traditional healers there to exchange information.

If possible, try to let people know of your visit in advance

Your journey will be wasted if the people you want to see are not at home.

Always follow the same approach so as not to forget important information

You should begin by asking questions concerning:

- first: the mother
- second: the children; newborn, preschool, schoolchildren
- third: the father and other adults
- fourth: possible diseases
- fifth: the environment.

What to take with you on your visits

(1) Take a simple first-aid kit and soap. This can be very useful for any emergency you might meet.

(2) Take a notebook to remind you whom to see and what to take. Your note might look like this:

Beku village   Amos – TB tablets?
                      Sanu – very small new baby. FP?

This will remind you: (1) to take extra TB tablets in case Amos has run out of them; (2) to talk to Sanu's parents about birth spacing, and to take pills and condoms to show them.

The notebook is also useful for recording health facts and problems you have found out, for example, from the traditional birth attendant, the traditional healer, the health committee, and by talking to people and looking around. This will help you when you next meet with the health service staff for discussion and also in reporting to your community committee.

Wherever possible, visit first the families who have no infections

This is important. This will reduce the risk of your carrying infection from one house to another. See people in the following order:

- first: mothers with new babies

- second: families (for discussions or demonstrations)

- third: visits to people with T B, colds, infectious diseases.

Recording your home visits

(1) Add *any new information* about births, deaths, or sicknesses to your charts or records.

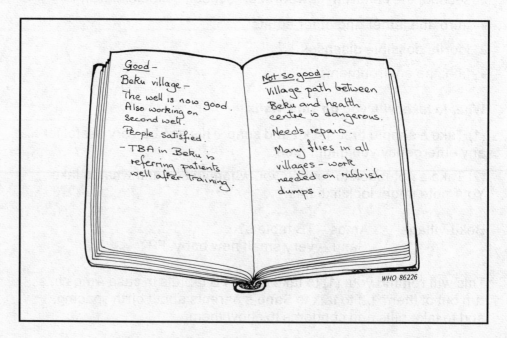

WHO 86226

(2) Make a note in your diary about any house *you should visit again* in one or two months.

(3) List the things you have seen (good and not so good) which you want *to talk about* at the next meeting of the community committee.

Unit 47

Getting active support from people [1]

You can help your community to improve its health only if
the people want you to help them. You should not impose
yourself on people. You have to win their support.

You should help people to do things you wish them to do
and you should not do yourself what they must do.

Learning objectives

After studying this unit you should be able to:

1 Explain to people why you must have their support in your health
   work.

2 Organize activities in order to get the people's support.

3 Give examples to the community of different types of support
   they may give you.

4 Discuss with community leaders what actions should be taken to
   solve health problems of the community, and take part in the
   meetings of community committees to provide information and to
   make suggestions to help *them* to make decisions.

---

[1] See also *On being in charge: a guide for middle-level management in primary
health care.* Geneva, World Health Organization, 1980.

You need help from the people in your work

The health problems described in this book must have given you an idea of how much work there is to do in a community. It is clear that *you cannot do all of it by yourself*, and you should not try to do so. The people themselves must do much of this work. When people work for themselves they value it more, and they quickly learn how to do more.

In Unit 1 you identified those who will work with you to improve health, namely:

- members of the "community development committee"

- groups such as women's groups, religious groups, scouts, workers' unions, and Red Cross or Red Crescent workers

- other men and women in the community who are willing to help.

The people know that the community committee makes the decisions and suggestions and gets the people to take action. Thus, it is best if the committee, and not you, makes decisions about health action. You can give committee members the information they need about health matters and you can suggest different things that men, women, children, families, or the whole community might do. When the committee members meet, they will discuss the information and suggestions you have given them and decide what needs to be done, how it may be done, and who will do it. If the committee members trust you, they will probably ask for your advice again.

Sometimes the work (for example, cleaning a street or digging a latrine) may be done best and most quickly by small groups of people in their own localities (say 3–10 families). The people in such small groups know one another well and are therefore more likely to work together to improve health. How to form small action groups is best decided at a meeting of the whole community. Other work, such as laying pipes for a water supply, would need the help of several small groups working together, or each doing different bits of the whole job.

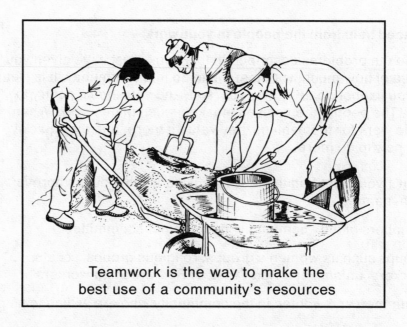

Teamwork is the way to make the
best use of a community's resources

Each group should agree on one person who will be its leader. This
person's name should be made known to the whole community.
When a community committee decides about action to be taken, it
is these group leaders who will find a way of doing it in their small
household groups (blocks or compounds). Arrange to meet these

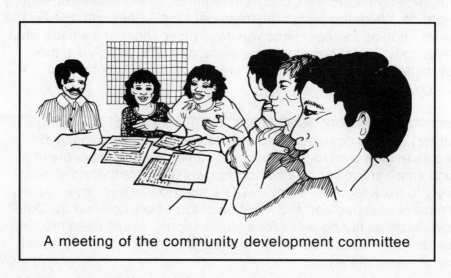

A meeting of the community development committee

leaders individually or in groups as often as *they* feel that they need to talk with you.

A community committee should meet at least 4 times a year and more often if necessary. Give its members information about the health of the community whenever you meet them. The committee may want to meet more often if you tell them about some problem that needs a quick decision and early action. You will be better informed if you have weekly meetings with the group leaders.

How to get people to help you

People will be eager to act and will support you if:

- You help in matters that concern them. For instance, if they feel that mosquitos are more of a nuisance than diarrhoea, help them to deal with the mosquito problem first.

- You help them to identify something they can do to improve their life and health without outside help, whenever possible.

- You link health actions to other activities of the community. For example, if an irrigation scheme is to be started, it would not take much effort or money to provide safe drinking-water at the same time. If fields are being drained to improve agriculture, swamps where mosquitos breed could be drained at the same time.

- You encourage the committee to set targets. For example, "by the end of next month every group leader will have listed the name and age of every person in each house in his block, and have given the health worker the name of every pregnant woman". When the target has been reached, suggest that the community makes a celebration and then sets a new target.

- You record what has been done for all to see, and especially for the community committee.

Different ways in which the community can support health activities

Other types of support or action by the community include, for example:

Setting up a fund

A special community health fund is useful. The committee will decide how to start and manage it. It could be used for:

- buying essential equipment, tools or medicines

- digging, protecting, or maintaining wells

- setting up a cooperative shop that will sell such essential items as razor blades for the delivery kit, condoms, aspirins, and sticking plaster

- paying for transport of sick persons to the health centre or hospital in an emergency

- buying petrol for the health worker's motor cycle.

Together with the community you can probably think of many more uses for such a community fund.

Using unused land to produce more food

Land that is not being used or not being used well can be used to raise funds. The community may work together on a piece of land given (or bought) for the benefit of the community, for example, to

- grow food for weaning babies, or extra food for preschool children, or meals for all schoolchildren

- raise cows or goats to provide extra milk for pregnant women, the sick, and the elderly

- grow a cash crop, which then can be sold to set up a community benefit fund for making a road or a well, for example.

Using local skills and resources for the benefit of the community

Every community has people with a wide range of skills and resources that can help in a number of ways to improve community life and health, and to support you in your health work. For example:

■ The local school with the help of the teacher could make a map of the community, its food and water resources, its swamps and unhealthy areas.

■ The teacher might be willing to help you prepare your monthly records for the health centre.

■ The teacher might encourage school competitions in making health posters to pin up in your health unit or in public places in the village.

■ The local religious leader might be asked if he would make a list of the health actions decided by the community committee,

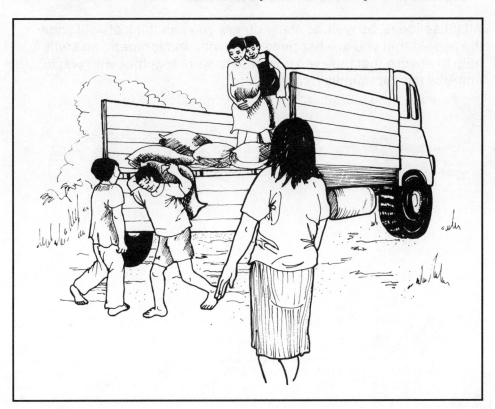

and the target dates, so that he can remind the people about them at religious services.

- The shopkeeper might help to keep the accounts of the health fund.

- The shopkeeper might increase stock to include basic health supplies such as sticking-plaster, aspirins, razor blades for the delivery kit, sugar and salt for the treatment of diarrhoea, and contraceptives.

- The scales that are used for weighing crops might also be used for weighing people, especially small children.

- Transport used by the people to take produce to market can be used to bring back from the market or from the health centre, supplies and equipment needed for health care.

All these ideas, as well as many others you can think of, will show the people that you are happy to work with and for them, and will help to ensure that they will continue to work together with you to improve the community's health.

Deciding what is urgent [1]

A community health worker will have to deal with certain problems immediately (an accident, a delivery, etc.), but most of the time there will be time to organize the work in order to be as useful as possible to the community.

Learning objectives

After studying this unit you should be able to:

1 Decide whether a problem is urgent and needs your immediate attention before anything else.

2 Discuss with the community committee and agree with it on the health problems that you must deal with first.

3 Agree with the community committee which health work the community will do.

4 Work out with your supervisor, and the community leaders, a plan for your work.

---

[1] See also *On being in charge: a guide for middle-level management in primary health care.* Geneva, World Health Organization, 1980.

Your job description

When the community committee and your supervisor have agreed on what can be done by you, they should first provide you with a job description (see Unit 49) so that you know clearly what you are expected to do. If you are not sure about some of your responsibilities, discuss the matter with your supervisor and clarify any uncertain points. You will then be able to organize and plan your own work.

In whichever way you plan your work, some problems will always arise that you will have to deal with immediately. This means that you will have to postpone some of the less urgent work.

What you must do immediately

What you must always do, before any other task, is to treat and attend to people who are dangerously sick, or injured in an accident, and need care urgently.

These are emergencies. You must stop everything else in order to help. The main problems that need care urgently are:

- heavy or continuous bleeding (see Unit 32)
- a severe pain in the belly (see Unit 28)
- burns on a large part of the skin (see Unit 30)
- a woman in labour (see Unit 16)
- diarrhoea and dehydration in a child (see Unit 26)
- severe headache with a stiff neck (see Unit 27)
- unconsciousness (see Unit 32)
- snake bites (see Unit 34)
- fractures (see Unit 33).

Note: This list is not in order of priority.

In all of these cases you must:

- try to get the patient to a health centre or hospital at once

- decide what you should do quickly in each case (see the Unit concerned) before the patient's departure for hospital.

Another emergency occurs when several or many people get sick at about the same time with vomiting, diarrhoea, belly pains, and fever. You must see them and treat them if necessary, and you must also try to find out what food or drink they have all had and try to stop other people from having the same food or drink until your supervisor says it is safe (see Unit 2).

Yet another emergency is when there is a natural disaster,[1] such as a fire, a flood, or an earthquake. Then there is a great danger that the water supply will break down and that the water will become dangerous to drink. Also, there may be many injured people. You must try to get help from the health centre and through your community leaders.

To be able to deal with these emergencies, you must:

- let the people know where you can be found
- keep ready for use a supply of medicines (including oral rehydration salts) and dressings
- work out with the community a reliable way of sending a message to your supervisor and the health centre or hospital
- work out with the community a reliable way of sending very sick and badly injured patients to hospital.

Work you must do regularly

Be available at special times in the day to treat sick people and to show them how to take care of themselves.

Visit people who are not sick but whose health needs to be watched. These include pregnant women, babies, other young children, and poor families. Give them as much information as they need in order to stay as well as possible.

---

[1] See also *WHO emergency health kit; standard drugs and clinic equipment for 10 000 persons for 3 months*. Geneva, World Health Organization, 1984.

Teach the people how to have good health and show them by your family's and your own example.

Do the work that you have agreed with the community committee or supervisor to do during a particular week or month.

To be able to do the above health work:

- You should make it known to everybody on which days of the week and at what times you will be at your post and where you can be found at other times.

- You should be at your health post at the time that you agree with your community committee or your supervisor.

- You should have a supply of medicines and dressings (see Annex 1).

- You should keep your records up to date so that you know which families and which problems need your special attention (see Unit 51).

- The community committee should be able to tell you whom you can call on for help when you need it.

What the community and families must do, with your help

The community and families must help to keep the environment clean and healthy (see Chapter 2) and improve the standard of living of the people.

- Make sure that every section of the community has a safe water supply and that it is kept safe.

- Help poor families, especially those with children, to have enough good and clean food, and to make the best use of the food they can get.

- Have a safe way of getting rid of excreta and other waste and make sure that all households use it.

- Have a reliable way of getting sick people to the health centre and hospital.

- Have a reliable way of sending messages to, and receiving messages from, the health centre and hospital.

In order that the community and families can do their health work:

- You must report regularly to the community committee about the health problems you find in the community.

- You must visit households in the community regularly, especially those with young children and those in which entire families are at risk. In this way you will know what their problems are and you will be able to discuss those problems with the households and advise them on how to deal with them.

- You may also have to suggest that the community committee invite the people to take an active part in tasks that have been agreed upon, such as those mentioned above.

Work out a plan for your work

Whenever possible, take advantage of the visit of your supervisor, for instance, at the beginning of the year, to have a joint meeting with the community leaders. At this meeting you can:

- review together the situation and the main problems in your community

- select together the problems you should deal with first

- decide together what action should be taken in the case of each problem selected, how long it should take, and how it should be done.

This will enable you to organize your work and plan your activities. It will also be a good way of letting everyone know what you are going to do during the coming months.

Unit 49

Knowing your work clearly [1]

The work of community health workers varies greatly from one country to another, depending on local conditions.

Health work is team work. Community health workers are members of health teams. They work in the community, with the help of the community leaders and services, but they cannot do everything and must refer the problems they cannot solve locally to the health centre or hospital.

Learning objectives

After studying this unit you should be able to:

1 Describe to your supervisor your work in detail.

2 Indicate what you cannot do and must refer to the health centre or hospital.

---

[1] See also *On being in charge: a guide for middle-level management in primary health care,* World Health Organization, Geneva, 1980.

What is your job description

Your job description is a description of the main activities you are expected to carry out as a CHW. This description should be agreed upon, on the basis of the needs of the community, by both the community leaders and your supervisor. It can be revised when necessary at their request, or at your own request if you think something should be changed in it. Here, as an illustration, is an example of a job description:

Job title: Community Health Worker (CHW) for District X.

Date: 1 January 1985.

Job summary: To care for the health of the community members, to maintain regular contact with the community leaders and the supervisor from the health services, to promote and take part in community projects.

Duties: 1. Primary health care activities. The CHW will give advice to anyone who comes to see him. He will give special care to those who have or may have the following diseases or conditions: malaria, diarrhoea, respiratory diseases, measles, wounds, burns, abscesses, skin diseases, malnutrition, venereal disease, eye infection, poisonous bites and stings, and intestinal worms. He will refer to the Medical Assistant of Y all complicated cases and those suspected of having any of the following diseases: TB, sleeping sickness, leprosy.

    2. Health promotion activities. Together with the Community Nurse and Midwife and other community workers, he will organize health education activities: discussions with mothers of young babies on immunization, oral rehydration in case of diarrhoea, good nutrition, and food. He will advise the community about water supply, waste disposal, use of latrines.

    3. He will report and keep records of his work and events happening in the community, according to specific instructions.

    4. He is responsible for the proper maintenance of his health post and the safe custody and renewal of its equipment, essential drugs, and supplies.

    5. He will attend refresher training sessions as announced.

Relations: The CHW reports to both the community committee and the Medical Assistant in charge of Y, who will appraise his work every year.

This job description is an important document because it tells you what you have to do. The training you will follow will prepare you to carry out the activities listed in it, and will help you to solve the problems you will be facing.

Sometimes there are two community health workers, a woman and a man, in the same community. In this case, the work can be shared; for instance the woman may do most of the health care work with the women and children, and the man may deal mostly with health work outside the household, such as water and food safety and keeping the environment healthy. Both will share the care of the sick.

As a CHW you must always remember that you are a member of a team of health workers. Although you may be alone in the community, you must keep in touch with the other members of the health team in the health centre. In this way, you will be able to keep them informed about your problems and call on them for help when you need it. You will also be able to increase your own knowledge and skills as a health worker.

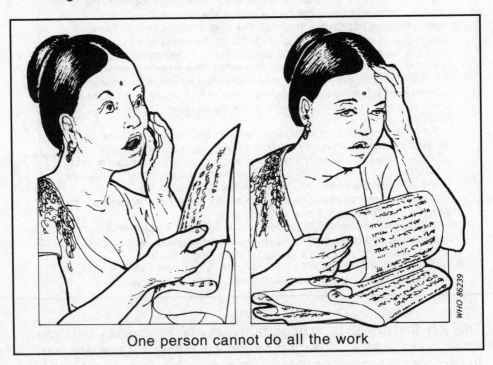

One person cannot do all the work

What you cannot do and have to refer

You have learned from this book that there are some problems that you can treat but there are certain others that you cannot, and those you must refer to the health centre or hospital for care by a nurse, midwife, or doctor. Sometimes the problem you refer to the health centre will be an emergency, and you should refer your patient at once, having first quickly provided first aid. At other times the referral may not be as urgent. At yet other times, you may need to ask your supervisor or another health worker to come to see a patient at home. You should try to get to know well the other health workers,

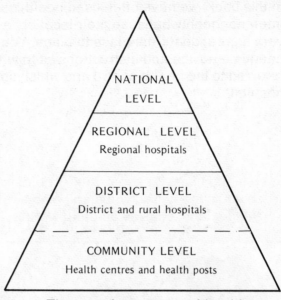

The usual structure of health services in a country

especially in the health centre, to whom you send patients. You should discuss your problems with them, and they should send you information that will help you to look after patients they have seen.

As we have seen, you should work out with the community leaders reliable ways of sending messages and patients to your supervisor as well as to the health centre or hospital.

There will also be another type of health problem that you may not be able to deal with. For example, if you are a woman, it may be that men will not like to come to you with certain problems. If you come to know of such problems you should arrange for a male health worker to come and see the man. If you are a man, it will sometimes happen that a woman patient, or a pregnant woman, may not want to discuss her problems with you. You must then ask a woman health worker to see her.

In this book, we have often used health centres and hospitals interchangeably because their location, availability, or equipment vary a great deal from place to place. Your supervisor will give you adequate advice and instructions as to which cases should be referred to the health centre and which should be sent direct to the hospital.

Unit 50

Equipment and supplies [1]

To do your job properly and well you need some basic equipment and supplies so that you can:

- *visit families and community groups*
- *treat patients*
- *record and report data and activities*
- *ask for help when needed.*

What you can get will depend on the resources available and what you are allowed to do.

The community will provide most of the equipment and supplies. The health services may provide some through your supervisor.

Equipment and supplies must be properly kept and stored.

Learning objectives

After studying this unit you should be able to:

1 Identify and indicate to your supervisor what equipment and supplies you need.

2 Decide to whom you must make the request for supplies and equipment and make the request in writing.

3 Explain how to keep and store the equipment and supplies.

---

[1] See: *WHO emergency health kit: standard drugs and clinic equipment for 10 000 persons for 3 months.* Geneva, World Health Organization, 1984, and *On being in charge: a guide for middle-level management in primary health care.* Geneva, World Health Organization, 1980.

The equipment and supplies you need for your work

At a health post the least you need is:

- a covered place, or room, with a sign indicating that it is a health post

- a table and two chairs

- one or two benches

- one cupboard that you can lock.

More space and furniture will help you and your visitors to be more comfortable.

There should be a proper light at all times. Near the health post clean water and latrines should be available. The latrines should be kept very clean.

Non-technical equipment and supplies for the health post

- 1 or 2 pans, bowls and glasses or cups

- 1 or 2 washbasins

- 1 or 2 containers for clean water

- soap, towels, a nail brush (for cleaning nails)

- a broom, a bucket, sponges, dusters

- scissors, knives, spoons

- alcohol

- a few notebooks, pencils and pens, a ruler

- if possible, a small spirit burner, or means of making a fire for sterilizing equipment.

Technical equipment and supplies for the health post

A standard list of equipment has probably been agreed upon by the health services. Check with your supervisor. It will include:

- thermometers

- cotton wool and dressings

- bandages and sticking plaster

- drugs (special list for community health workers) (see also Annex 1)

- forms for reporting and ordering drugs and supplies (see Unit 52)

- possibly, syringes and needles.

A bicycle

This is not essential but may be useful if your community is spread over a large area. It may be the only means of contacting your supervisor.

Who to write to for supplies and how to make your requests

Since you are a community health worker, it is mainly from the community that you will obtain the non-technical material (chairs, cupboards, bowls, etc.) for your work. However, the health services may provide some of the technical equipment, particularly drugs, depending on local policies and organization.

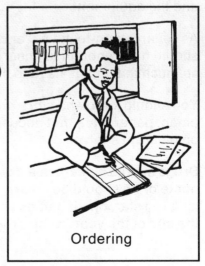

Ordering

You should send your request to the community leader and your technical supervisor when your stock is getting low.

Requests should be made, if possible, in writing and handed to the community leader or your supervisor. Follow the instructions you have received. If you have not received any instructions or a supply of order forms, you can make your request as follows:

Mr (name of supervisor or community leader)   Date: 28 May 1985
  Please send me:
    soap, 10 bars
    pencils, 2
    iodine solution 2.5%, 6 bottles
    cotton wool, 6 packets
  which I will need during the next three months.
    With all my thanks,
      XXX (your name and address)
      Community Health Worker.

How to keep and store equipment and supplies

You should always keep your health post clean and pleasant for the people who come to you. If necessary, ask the community leaders to help you to maintain it in good condition and to carry out the work needed in connection with the post itself, the furniture and the equipment.

As regards non-technical and technical equipment or supplies, you should have enough to ensure that you do not run short, but not so much that things have to be thrown away.

You should *keep and store drugs* separately from other supplies (soap, paper, etc.), not necessarily in another cupboard but at least on different shelves.

Drugs should be kept in a dry, cool place away from light. Each bottle or tin should be clearly labelled. Stick a special mark, such as a red star, on all bottles or drugs that should be used before the end of the year. Keep drugs in a locked cupboard.

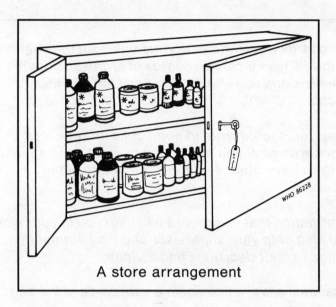

A store arrangement

Note: The upper shelf to be used first. The stars show drugs that expire this year.

Unit 51
Keeping records

Health records are written information about the health of the people. These include: records of births and deaths, illnesses, pregnancies, immunizations, and sanitary conditions.

Each day you should write in notebooks, in registers, or on forms or cards what you have done or what has happened or what you have observed about the health of the community.

The information that you record will help you in your work and will also help your supervisor and the community committee in their decisions and actions.

Records must always be kept in a safe place at the health post.

Learning objectives

After studying this unit you should be able to:

1 Explain why you should record information.

2 Tell what information you need to record.

3 Obtain information about the people's health and the effects of your health care activities.

4 Keep simple records accurately.

5 Record in a standard form

  ■ births and deaths that have occurred in your community

  ■ people's illnesses and your health care activities

  ■ all other actions you have taken to improve the health of the community.

Why you have to keep simple records

Only some information can be kept in your head, for example, who are the most influential members of the community or when are the market days.

You will not always remember details, for example, which children have already had measles or which children have been immunized.

Once obtained, information should not be lost. Therefore, it should be recorded.

In Unit 52 "Preparing and writing reports", you will see that you must regularly give your supervisor and your community committee information you have obtained in order to enable them to make decisions and take action. The records you keep will help you in doing this.

The information contained in your records will also help you:

- To know and remember the babies, mothers, and other persons you have seen or have to follow up, what you advised them to do last time you saw them (for example, what immunizations they should have and when and where to go for them), or what progress, if any, has taken place since you last saw a particular patient.

- To decide what action to take (for instance, if you have noted several cases of the same disease in the last few days, you will have to inform your supervisor and the community leaders).

- To remember the problems you would like to discuss at the next meeting of the community committee or during your supervisor's next visit.

- To prepare your reports or to order the drugs you need in good time.

- To plan future activities and to decide on what matters you need to get advice from your supervisor.

- To recall important events in your community, in particular births and deaths.

What information do you need to record?

To do good work, you will need to have information about:

- *the community* (population, maps, health needs, names of the members of the community committee, activities planned to help the development of the community) (see Unit 1)

- the important events that take place in the community, in particular *births and deaths*

- what has been done to improve the health of the people: *immunizations* (see Unit 21), health education, family planning (Unit 18)

- the *illnesses* that people have, and what treatment or care they are getting

- the *drugs* and *supplies* that you get, store, distribute, and keep in stock.

Your supervisor will advise you on the details you need to know to keep good and simple records.

How can you get the information you need?

The members of the community know most of the information you need to record:

- *Listen* to what they say about their health and *ask* them what you need to know, for example, what problems they have, what they need to improve their health, or whether there is a pregnant woman or a newborn baby in the family.

- *Look at* things that are important for the health of the people, for example, wells and latrines. Are they safe? Are they used properly? Do they need to be improved?

- *Check* and *count* things or events so that you will know how many there are and can decide what to do. For example, if there are more than the usual number of cases of diarrhoea in one week, you must notify your supervisor. If your supply of aspirin tablets is running out, you must order a new supply.

How to keep simple records

The method of recording information differs from country to country.

Some of the information can be kept in *individual* records (i.e., a record card for each person). For example, you can record a child's weight on a growth chart. Other information can be recorded in *family* registers: you or the father or mother can note, for example, dates of birth, dates of immunizations, serious illnesses, and other events of health interest. Families can keep these records and registers in their homes.

The family or you can also enter in this book the date on which something to be remembered happened, and a very short description of what happened. A household book may look like this:

```
Date

1.6.1980      Ely's left wrist broken
8.8.1981      Baby boy born: Fred!
11.9.1981     Health inspector
                checked tube-well
etc.
```

In some countries, special cards or books have been printed for households to record health problems and immunizations. The names and dates of birth of all the members of a family or household are listed, together with the main health events. Ask your supervisor whether this is being done anywhere in your country.

Whatever the method being used in your country, remember that *you* will need to record most of the information and keep it up to date in a register, notebook, or diary. You must keep it in a safe place so that other people cannot see it.

Recording

The following formats are *examples* of ways of recording births, deaths, illnesses, and health activities. The health service in your country may be using a different form, particularly for immunization (see Unit 21). Ask your supervisor about it.

(1) *Information about births*. This may be recorded in columns in a register or copybook as follows:

Date of birth	Name of child	Sex[1] M/F	Names and address of parents	Name of person assisting with birth	Child born alive? Yes/No	Weight of child at birth

[1] M = male, F = female

(2) *Deaths may be recorded* with information written in columns in a register or notebook, as follows:

Date of death	Name of dead person	Sex M/F	Age	Probable cause of death	Name of person reporting death

(3) *Illnesses and what you do to treat them*. This information must be recorded in an *illness register*, or better, on a separate card or page for each person.

From the illness register you will know what kinds of illnesses there are in the community, and which people need special attention.

The information may be written in columns in a notebook or register, as follows:

Date	Name and address of patient	Age	Sex M/F	Complaint	CHW's findings	Action taken	Notes

(4) *Other activities*. It is very useful to make notes every day about what you have done, particularly about those actions that the community committee or your supervisor should know about and those that must be followed up.

You will need a diary in which you should note daily information on:

- health education and advice given
- action taken to improve sanitation and cleanliness in the homes and village
- private meetings held with local authorities
- meetings of village committee
- other events or activities of importance to your work.

A page of your diary may look like this:

Monday 1 November
Visited Segano hamlet
Met with Committee Chairman. Must tell him date of next immunization session

Tuesday 2 November
Visited Pelo hamlet
Inform district about lack of spare parts for tube-well

Wednesday 3 November
Talked with women's club about making dish racks. At next meeting ask how many made and discuss different designs.

> ### Remember!
>
> If you have not got a separate notebook and diary, one notebook can be divided into sections to record the different types of information.
>
> You keep and use records to help you in your work.
>
> If you keep good records of information your work will become easier and better.

Unit 52

Preparing and writing reports

Your reports are the information you write and send to your supervisor and your community committee to show what important things you have seen, what you have done about the health of the community, and what you have recorded in your notebooks.

You should discuss your reports with the community committee and with your supervisor.

The information given in reports, how often they are written, and how they are used, will differ from country to country. The two formats in this chapter are only examples and should be adapted to the needs of different health services.

You must send your reports on time and you must keep a copy of each report in a safe place at the health post.

The names of patients should not be written in reports.

Learning objectives

After studying this unit you should be able to:

1 Prepare and write a health report and a medicines and supplies report.

2 State what you should expect from the community and your supervisor in return for the information you give them.

Using records to prepare reports

When required to do so (for instance, on the last day of each month), you should use your records to prepare 2 reports:

(1) *A health report* containing the following information:

- number of births

- number of deaths

- kinds and numbers of illnesses or injuries

- your other health activities

- your comments

- comments of the community committee.

This information could be written as shown opposite.

Under item 7, the community health worker should write what he thinks the community committee or his supervisor should know, for instance, the probable causes and the circumstances of the deaths that have occurred, and whether the community health worker thinks the deaths could have been prevented.

(2) *A drugs and supplies report*, containing the following information:

- name of the item (medicine, soap, cotton wool, etc.)

- amount in stock on the first day of the month

- amount received during the month

- amount used during the month

- amount remaining

- amount needed for the next supply.

HEALTH REPORT FOR THE COMMUNITY OF————————————————
YEAR ———— MONTH ———————— NAME OF CHW ——————————————

1. Number of births (during the month):
    - ———————— males born alive
    - ———————— females born alive
    - ———————— born dead
    - ———————— TOTAL BIRTHS

2. Number of deaths (during the month):
    - ———————— under 5 years old
    - ———————— 5 years old and over
    - ———————— TOTAL DEATHS

3. Number of patients seen (during the month):
    - ———————— under 5 years old
    - ———————— 5 years old and over
    - ———————— TOTAL PATIENTS SEEN

4. Number of patients sent to the health centre or hospital:
    - ————————

5. Number of complaints (during the month):[1]
    - ———————— fever   ———————— burns
    - ———————— diarrhoea   ———————— malnutrition
    - ———————— wounds   ———————— others

6. Other CHW health activities: ————————————————————————
    ——

7. CHW comments:——
    ——
    ——
    ——
    ——

                                              Signature ——————————————

                    *   *   *   *   *   *   *   *

Community Committee comments: ————————————————————————————

Supervisor comments: ————————————————————————————————————

[1] The health services in each country will use their own special lists of complaints, appropriate to the local situation.

371

This information could be written in a form such as:

Item[1] A	In stock on first day of month B	Received during the month C	Amount used during month D	Remaining at the end of the month E $(=B+C-D)$	Amount requested for next supply F

Drugs and supplies report for the community of _____
Year _____ Month _____ Name of CHW_____

[1] A standardized list of medicines and supplies can be used if desired. Also other items such as soap, bricks, bags of cement, etc.

The number written in column B should be the same as the number written in column E of the previous month's report.

Note: Some health services may find it convenient to have their reporting forms printed and distributed in advance to the community health workers in order to standardize information. If this is done, it could be helpful to have the forms printed in three different colours: one colour to be kept at the health post, one colour for the community committee, and one colour for the supervisor. In that case, the community health worker must prepare three copies of his report.

Discussing reports with the community committee

The CHW should discuss the health report and drugs and supplies report at the community committee meeting. The committee

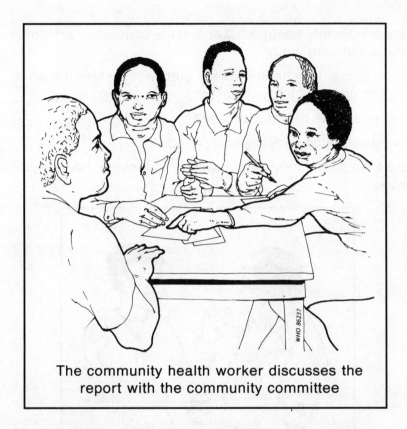

The community health worker discusses the
report with the community committee

members will then know what the problems are and what the
community needs to do to solve those problems. From the reports
they will be able to:

- know what the community health worker does

- discuss how they can help him in his work

- comment on the report

- decide on any action that needs to be taken in the community.

Discussing the reports with the supervisor

The CHW should also discuss the reports with his supervisor. His
supervisor will then know the state of health of the community and

373

what the community health worker and the committee are doing. Then the supervisor can:

- give the community health worker guidance on how the work should be done, which kinds of problems to refer, etc.

- advise what else needs to be done

- see what supplies and drugs are needed

- discuss the community health worker's plans for the next period of work.

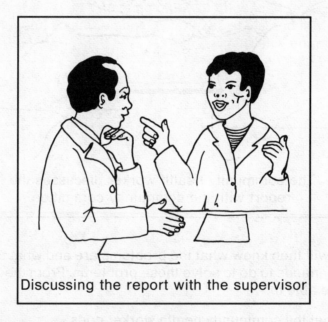

Discussing the report with the supervisor

In return for the information you supply to the community and to your supervisor, what should you expect?

From the community

A community can take an active part in protecting its own health when its leaders and the people understand well:

- their own health needs

- what can be done about them

- how well things are being done to improve health.

You are in a good position to help the community to understand these three points. If you do this well, the community will take an active part in health care. People will also give you better information about themselves when they see that you are using this information for their benefit.

From the supervisor

You should expect his strong support for your work. He will be able to respond better and faster to your requests if he receives regular reports. He will be able to see that you know what is happening, and therefore he will trust you more.

Annexes

Medicines [1]

How to give them, how much to give

Ask your supervisor to tell you the local names (if any) given to these medicines in your country; these may be easier to remember and spell than the scientific names.

Some general information

Remember that:

(1) The dosage of medicine is different for a baby under one year old, a small child (1–3 years old), a child (4–12 years old) and an adult (or a child over 12).

(2) Medicines may be given in different ways:

- by injection
- as tablets
- in drops
- in liquid or ointment form for putting on the skin
- in powder form.

(3) Medicines will cure people only if they are given in the proper way.

Injections. See Annex 2 for instructions on how to give injections.

Tablets. Adults can swallow tablets without any difficulty but babies cannot. For babies and children, crush the tablets into a powder and mix with fruit juice, treacle, or jam.

Drops. These are easy to give. Count the number of drops to be given.

---

[1] The term "medicine" is used in this annex interchangeably with the term "drug".

Liquids or ointments. Spread them on the skin with your fingers or with clean cotton wool.

Powders. Mix with water.

(4) The medicine may need to be given once or several times a day. When it is given several times a day, there should be an interval between each dose, for example, one tablet at 8 a.m., one at noon, one at 4 p.m. and one at 8 p.m.

(5) Use the list on the following pages only as instructed in the different units in this book.

(6) Never buy or use medicines that you do not know. This can be very dangerous.

(7) When used properly, medicines will enable you to treat most health problems in an effective and efficient way. However, remember that medicines are dangerous and costly. Therefore, they should be used carefully and should not be wasted. Always bear in mind that not all patients need medicines and that sometimes the best treatment is to let nature cure the problem. In all cases, it is better to give no medicine at all than to give the wrong medicine.

(8) It is your job to explain to the patient why and how he should take the medicine that has been prescribed.

Important remarks

(1) The names of the medicines given in this book are generic names. Each country should specify if it wishes to use different names.

(2) The dosages and the packaging may vary from one country to another. The list should therefore be revised to conform to local conditions.

1 tablet	⊘
1/2 tablet	⬭
1/4 tablet	◺

(3) All of the following medicines are listed in the revised model list of essential drugs published by WHO (WHO Technical Report Series, No. 722, 1985).

How to use the medicines mentioned in this book

Name of medicine	Used mainly for treatment of:	Form in which it is given	How much to give			
			Baby (less than 1 year old)	Small child (1–3 years)	Child (4–12 years)	Adult (or child over 12 years old)
Aluminium hydroxide	abdominal pains	500-mg tablets	—	—	—	1 tablet 4 times a day for 5 days
Aspirin	fever and pains	500-mg tablets	—	$\frac{1}{4}$ tablet 3 times a day	$\frac{1}{2}$ tablet 3 times a day	1–3 tablets 3 times a day
Benzoic + salicylic acid	skin diseases	ointment	First wash the skin with soap and water and leave to dry. Then put the ointment directly on the skin. Repeat once a day for 3 days.			
Benzyl benzoate	skin diseases (fungi)	liquid to put on the skin	First wash the skin with soap and water and leave to dry. Then put the liquid on the skin either directly or with a clean cloth. Repeat once a day for 3 days.			
Charcoal, activated	poisoning, abdominal pains	powder to be mixed with water	—	—	$\frac{1}{2}$ tablespoon 3 times a day	1 tablespoon 3 times a day
Chloroquine	fever (treatment of malaria)	150-mg tablets	$\frac{1}{2}$ tablet daily for 3 days	1 tablet daily for 3 days	3 tablets daily for 3 days	6 tablets daily for 3 days
Ergometrine	bleeding after delivery or miscarriage	0.2-mg tablets	—	—	—	1 or 2 tablets; repeat once or twice if necessary
Gentian violet or iodine (tincture)	cleaning wounds, skin diseases	liquid to put on skin	First wash the skin with soap and water and leave to dry. Then pour a few drops of the liquid on the wound or spread on the skin with a clean cloth			
Ipecacuanha	poisoning (to vomit poison)	Syrup to drink	—	$\frac{1}{2}$ tablespoon once	1 tablespoon once	2 tablespoons once
Iron sulfate (ferrous salt)	anaemia, weakness, tiredness	60-mg tablets	—	—	1 tablet to be taken with food once or twice a day for 1 month	
Mebendazole	intestinal worms (round worms, pinworms)	100-mg tablets	—	—	2 tablets to be taken with food twice a day for 3 days.	
Metronidazole	trichomoniasis	500-mg tablets	—	—	—	4 tablets once
Neomycin/ bacitracin ointment	skin diseases (infections)	ointment	First wash the skin with soap and water, and leave to dry. Then put the ointment on the skin with a clean cloth. Repeat once a day for 3 days			
Niclosamide	intestinal worms (flat worms, tape worms)	500-mg tablets	—	1 tablet once	2 tablets once	4 tablets once
Oral rehydration salts (ORS)	Diarrhoea	1 packet dissolved in 1 litre of drinking water	As much as is needed to quench thirst. Then 1–2 cupfuls for each watery stool passed. Adults may need several litres a day. Continue until diarrhoea stops.			

Name of medicine	Used mainly for treatment of:	Form in which it is given	How much to give			
			Baby (less than 1 year old)	Small child (1–3 years)	Child (4–12 years)	Adult (or child over 12 years old)
Penicillin	infections	Intramuscular injection				
■ procaine benzylpenicillin (medium-term effect)			—	250 000 units every day for 3 days	500 000 units every day for 3 days	1 000 000 units every day for 3 days
■ benzathine benzylpenicillin (long-term effect)			—	600 000 units once		1 200 000 units once
■ ampicillin (short-term effect)		500-mg tablets	—	—	4–8 tablets per day for 4 days (2–4 in the morning, 2–4 in the evening)	
Phenobarbital	to treat someone who has convulsions	50-mg tablets	—	$\frac{1}{2}$ tablet	1 tablet	1–2 tablets
				2 or 3 times a day for 2 days then half the dosage for 6 months		
Piperazine	intestinal worms (roundworms)	500-mg tablets	2 tablets once	3 or 4 tablets once	6 tablets once	8 tablets once
	very small worms	(crush to a powder, and mix with a sweet drink if necessary)	$\frac{1}{2}$ tablet 3 times a day for a week	1 tablet 3 times a day for a week	$1\frac{1}{2}$ tablets 3 times a day for a week	$1\frac{1}{2}$ tablets 3 times a day for a week
Retinol (vitamin A)	eye diseases	60-mg tablets (200 000 IU)	—	$\frac{1}{2}$ tablet once	1 tablet once	1 tablet once
Silver nitrate	eye diseases (newborn babies)	drops in the eyes	2 or 3 drops in the corner of the eye just after the delivery	—	—	—
Sulfamethoxazole + trimethoprim	infections	400 + 80-mg tablets	—	$\frac{1}{2}$ tablet twice a day for 5 days	1 tablet twice a day for 5 days	2 tablets twice a day for 5 days
Tetracycline	eye diseases	eye ointment	Put a little ointment ($\frac{1}{2}$ cm) in the corner of the eye 2–3 times a day for 3–5 days			
	infections	250-mg tablets	$\frac{1}{4}$ tablet 4 times a day for 3 days	$\frac{1}{2}$ tablet 4 times a day for 3 days	1 tablet 4 times a day for 3 days	1 to 3 tablets 4 times a day for 3 days
			Note: to be avoided, when possible, during pregnancy and in children under 8 years of age. Use ampicillin instead.			

Name of medicine	Used mainly for treatment of:	Form in which it is given	How much to give			
			Baby (less than 1 year old)	Small child (1–3 years)	Child (4–12 years)	Adult (or child over 12 years old)
Antivenom serum	snake bites	Injection	Requires a proper cold chain system. To be given only on your supervisor's instructions.			
Tetanus antitoxin (serum)	wounds, burns, to avoid getting tetanus	Injection	Requires a proper cold chain system. To be given with great caution only on your supervisor's instructions.			
Vaccines	to prevent infectious diseases	mostly given by injection	Requires a proper cold chain system. To be given only on your supervisor's instructions.			

Important techniques

1. Taking the temperature

There are three common ways of taking a person's temperature:
(a) by placing the thermometer in the mouth; (b) placing the
thermometer in the armpit; and (c) putting the thermometer in the
anus.

Taking temperature in the mouth or in the armpit

(1) Make sure that the column of mercury inside the thermometer
is below about 35 °C. If it is not, shake the thermometer until it
has gone down.

(2) Ask the patient to place the *small part* of the thermometer under
his tongue and keep his mouth closed, or in his armpit and hold
his elbow against his body.

(3) Leave the thermometer in place for about 2 minutes.

(4) Take the thermometer out and read the figure in line with the
top of the column of mercury inside the thermometer. If the figure
is above 37.5 °C the patient has a fever; the higher the figure, the
greater the fever.

(5) Clean the thermometer with some cotton wool and soapy water
(not hot water). Shake the thermometer so that the mercury goes
down towards the small part. Put the thermometer away so that it
does not fall on the ground and break.

Taking the temperature in the anus (see drawings on next page)

A different type of thermometer is used for taking anal temperature.
It has a rounded tip that will not damage the anus. You should *not*
use the same thermometer as you use for taking oral or armpit
temperatures.

(1) See that the line of mercury is below about 35 °C (see (1)
above).

(2) Ask the patient to push the *small part* of the thermometer into his anus. If the patient is a child or is unable to do it himself, you must insert it for him.

(3) Leave the thermometer in place for about 2 minutes. An adult should be lying on his side; a child (especially a small child) should lie on his stomach and you should hold him to prevent him from rolling over.

(4) Remove the thermometer and read the temperature as in step (4) above.

(5) Clean, shake down, and put away the thermometer as in step (5) above.

What temperatures do these thermometers show?

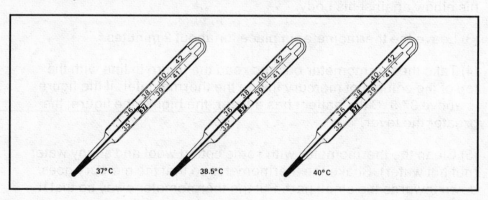

Note: If you do not have a thermometer, you can feel the temperature by placing your hand on the forehead of the patient and comparing its warmth with the warmth of your own forehead.

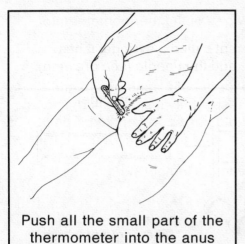

Push all the small part of the thermometer into the anus

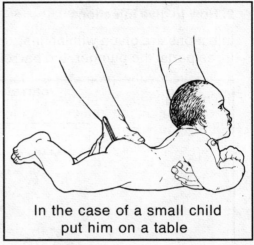

In the case of a small child put him on a table

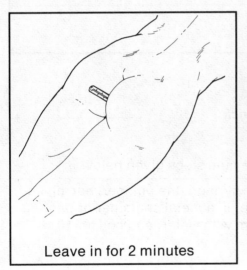

Leave in for 2 minutes

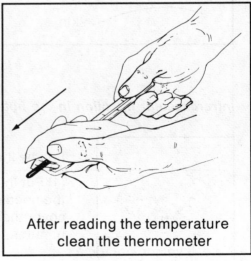

After reading the temperature clean the thermometer

2. How to give injections

Injections are given with an instrument called a syringe. It has three parts: the plunger, the barrel, and the needle (see drawing).

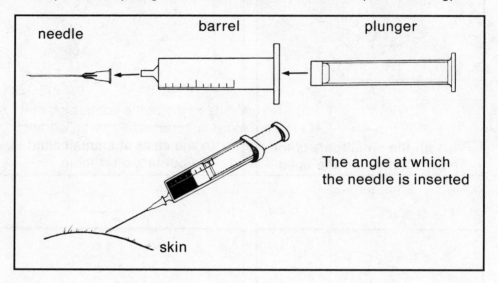

needle   barrel   plunger

The angle at which the needle is inserted

skin

Intramuscular injection in the buttock

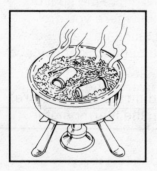

Follow the nine steps given below.

(1) Put the syringe (the plunger, barrel, and the needle) in a metal container or pan, cover them with water, and boil for 10 minutes.

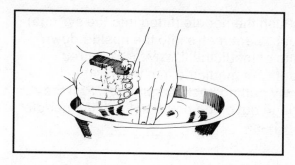

(2) Wash your hands well with soap and water.

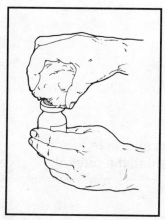

(3) Clean the lid of the bottle containing the medicine to be injected with a swab wetted with a disinfectant such as alcohol, iodine, or gentian violet. Rub hard 2–3 times.

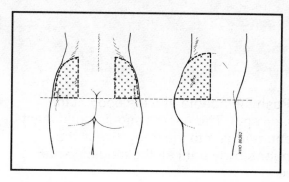

(4) With the same swab rub 2–3 times the spot on the skin where you are going to insert the needle. On the buttocks choose a place that is fairly high up and towards the side, as shown in the drawing.

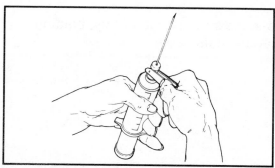

(5) Put the barrel and the plunger together and fit the needle firmly, holding it at its base (the end that is not pointed).

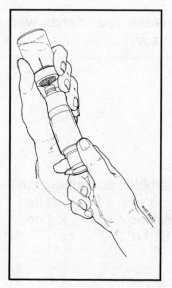

(6) Push the needle (fitted into the syringe) about 1 centimetre into the upside-down bottle of medicine. Draw the required quantity of medicine into the syringe by slowly pulling back the plunger. Pull the syringe out of the bottle holding the needle at its base.

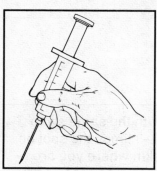

(7) Hold the syringe as shown in the drawing and stand behind the patient.

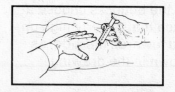

(8) Push the needle into the body at the chosen spot. The needle should go at least 2 centimetres into the body. Press the plunger slowly until all the medicine has gone in.

(9) Take the syringe out quickly, holding the needle at its base.

Subcutaneous injection (*in the arm or the forearm*)

Follow the instructions given for injection in the buttock (also see drawings).

Steps 1, 2, 3, 5 and *6*, are the same as for "Intramuscular injection" (in the buttocks) above.

Step 7. Hold the syringe as shown in the drawing below.

Step 8. Pick up the skin of the forearm (or the arm) with the fingers of your left hand. Push the needle into the skin which is pulled out, so that the needle goes in about one centimetre. Once the needle is under the skin, let go of the skin and press on the plunger of the syringe to make all the liquid go in. Pull the syringe and needle out, holding the needle at its base.

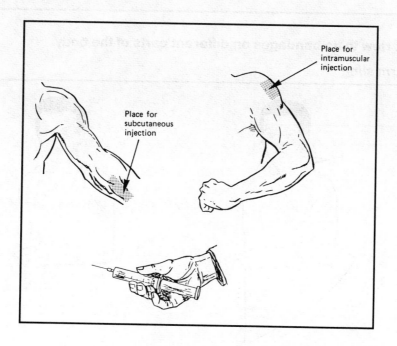

Place for intramuscular injection

Place for subcutaneous injection

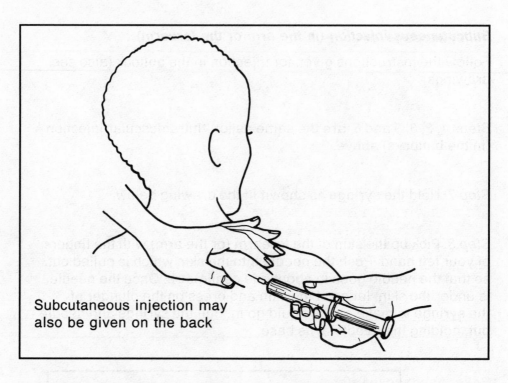

Subcutaneous injection may
also be given on the back

3. How to tie bandages on different parts of the body

Arm sling

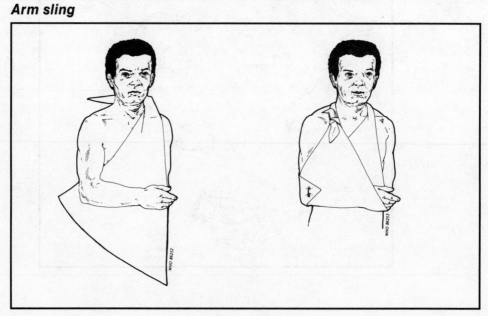

Roller bandage for upper arm

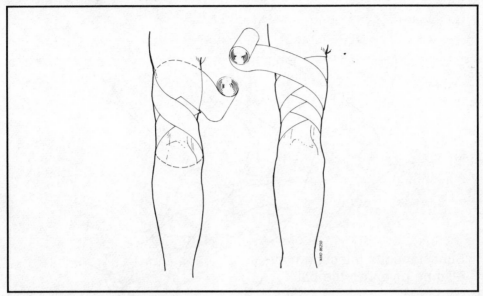

Roller bandage for elbow

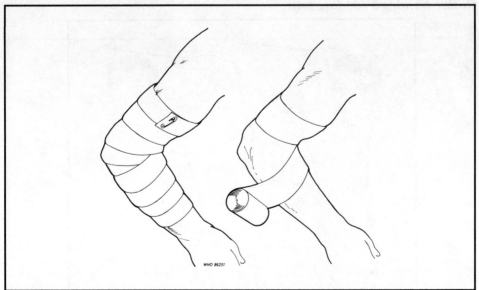

Elbow bandage

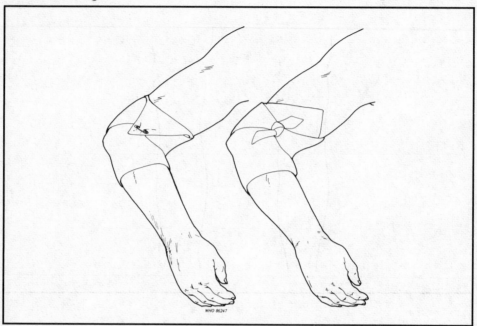

WHO 86247

Roller bandage for forearm

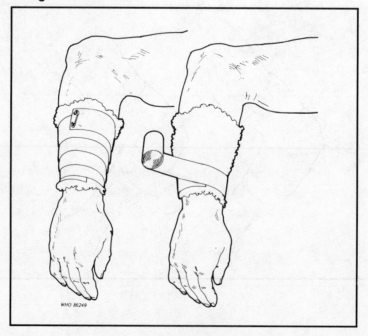

WHO 86249

394

Hand bandage

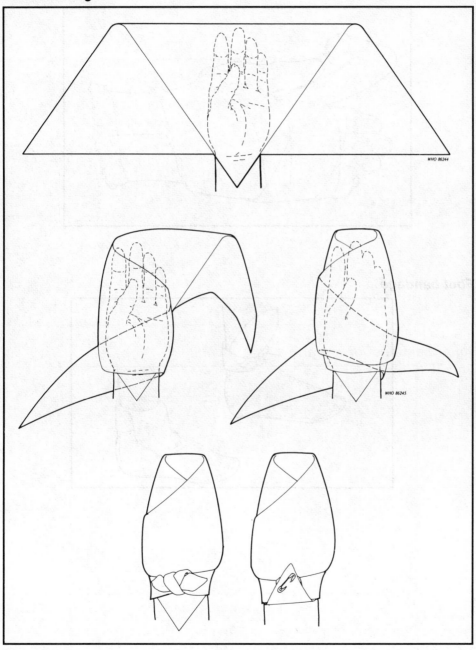

Roller bandage for hand

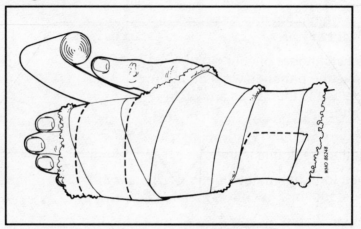

Foot bandage

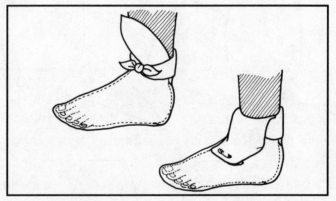

4. Counting the pulse

(1) Have a watch that has a second
hand in front of you.

(2) Place two fingers of your right
hand above the patient's wrist on the
same side as his thumb, as shown in
the drawing.

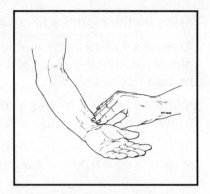

(3) Press very slightly. You should
feel a regular beat; this is the pulse.

(4) Count it for a full minute looking at your watch. The number of
beats you count in 1 minute is the *pulse rate*.

Normally it is between 70 and 80 beats per minute.

Pulse rate increases with:

- effort—so take the pulse when the patient has rested

- fever—38 °C = around 100
  39 °C = around 120

- dehydration—a pulse rate of 130 without fever may be a sign of
  severe dehydration

- some diseases of the heart.

5. How to give mouth-to-mouth resuscitation (artificial respiration)

If a newborn baby is not breathing but the heart is beating, he must
immediately be helped to breathe or he will die. The method
described below may also be used to help older children or adults
to breathe again if their breathing stops after falling into water or
after an electric shock, for instance.

For a newborn baby

(1) Clean the mouth, nose and throat quickly and gently to allow
air to pass easily into the chest.

(2) Lay the baby on his back with his head tilted back as indicated
in the illustration.

(3) Cover the mouth and nose with your mouth.

(4) Blow small breaths gently into the chest about 25–30 times a minute, so that the chest rises. Do not blow hard or you may harm the baby's chest.

(5) Pause to see if he has started breathing, and blow gently again. Continue to blow gently until the baby is breathing regularly.

(6) Air may pass into the child's belly. If you see the belly swell up, press on it from below to push the air out.

The baby may start breathing regularly almost at once, or you may have to continue to blow up his chest for about 15 minutes if the heart is still beating.

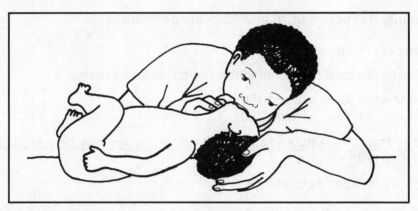

For an older child or adult

(1) Same as for a baby.

(2) Same as for a baby.

(3) Cover the patient's mouth with your own mouth, pulling up his lower jaw with one hand to clear the air passages to the chest.

(4) Blow air into the patient about 15–20 times a minute, using the full pressure of your chest to fill his. This means you take a deep breath and blow every 3 or 4 seconds.

(5) Lift your head and allow the air to escape, checking to see whether the patient has started to breathe. Continue until breathing starts. You may have to do it for more than one hour.

6. How to make a stretcher

(1) Take 2 sticks, each 2 metres long, and 2 shirts with their buttons fastened.

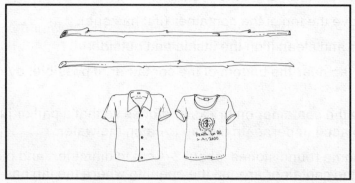

(2) Slip the sticks through the sleeves of the shirts as shown below.

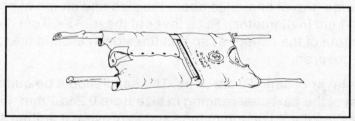

(3) The stretcher is ready. Now you can carry the patient comfortably to the hospital or health centre.

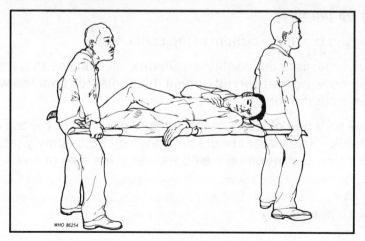

399

7. How to make and use a water filter (household size) [1]

Making the filter

(1) Get a barrel or any other container that is at least 1 metre deep.

(2) Remove the top of the container (if it has one).

(3) Scrub and clean it on the inside and outside.

(4) Fix a tap near the bottom of the container, if possible, by welding.

(5) Place the container on bricks or stones so that a pail or jug can be placed underneath the tap to catch the water.

(6) Get some round stones, about 2–4 cm in diameter, and place them in the container around the opening where the tap has been put. Place the stones in such a way that the opening to the tap is not blocked off completely.

(7) Get some gravel or stones about the size and shape of peas (about $\frac{1}{2}$–1 cm in diameter). Put a layer of these, 15–20 cm deep, in the bottom of the container so that the stones around the tap inlet are covered.

(8) Add a layer of sand 50 cm deep. The sand should be quite fine, with most of the particles ranging in size from 0.2 to 1 mm. Flat rocks may be placed on top of the sand to prevent it getting stirred up into the water.

Starting up the filter

(9) Close the tap at the bottom of the container.

(10) Pour water into the container. Do this carefully so that the sand at the top does not get stirred up. Fill the container until the water is 2–3 cm from the top.

(11) Draw off a pail of water at the tap and pour it into the top of the container. The water should be drawn off quite slowly (at a rate of about 1 litre per minute if the container is the size of an oil barrel).

---

[1] See Unit 4, "Water supply".

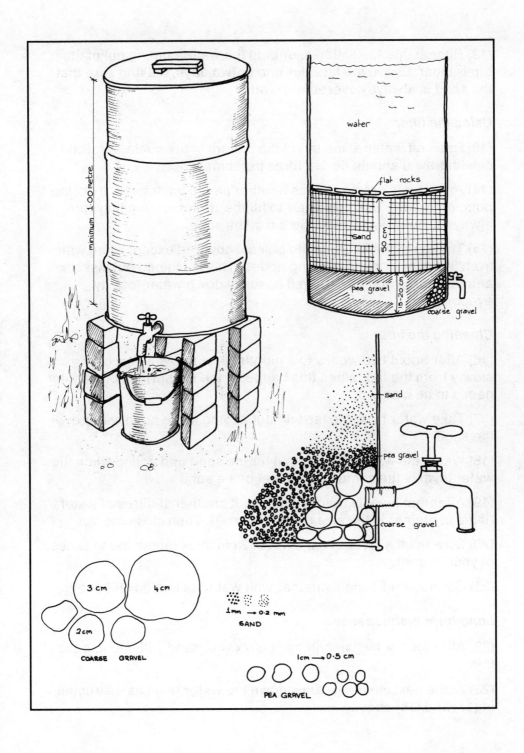

(12) Repeat this 15–20 times, or until the water coming out of the tap is clear. Leave the filter for one or two days, making sure that the sand is always covered with water.

Using the filter

(13) Draw off water at the tap at the bottom of the container. Rate of withdrawal should be 1–2 litres per minute.

(14) As water is drawn off, use another pail to fetch water from the pond or stream. Use this water to fill the container, making sure always to have water over the top of the sand.

(15) The top of the filter should be kept covered except when water from the river or pond is being added. This is to keep out insects, animals, birds and dirt, as well as to cut down water loss by evaporation.

Cleaning the filter

(16) After about two weeks to a month the water will flow only slowly from the tap. When this happens, the top surface of the filter needs to be cleaned.

(17) Take water from the tap without adding more pond water over the sand.

(18) Watch the water level drop over the sand and notice when the water level is the same as the level of the sand.

(19) After that level is reached, take out another 10 litres of water (if the container is the size of an oil barrel). Then close the tap.

(20) Scrape off a layer of sand about 2 cm thick (about the thickness of your thumb).

(21) Carefully refill the container with water as in step (10) above.

Long-term maintenance

(22) After four or five cleanings, the layer of sand will become too thin.

(23) At the next cleaning, draw down the water level as instructed in (17) and (18) above.

(24) Now take out about 25 litres of water so the water level is 10 cm below the surface of the sand. Save this water to put it back into the filter.

(25) Take out the sand down to the water level and save it in pails or gourds or a basket.

(26) Refill the filter with clean sand and then replace the sand you saved in (25) above as the top layer. Smooth the surface of the sand.

(27) The water you saved in (24) above should then be carefully poured back into the container.

(28) Fill the container with more water to within 2–3 cm of the top.

(29) Water taken from the tap should then be safe for drinking.

8. How to disinfect drinking-water with bleaching powder

Materials required

(1) A clean bottle of 1-litre capacity, preferably of brown or green coloured glass and having a tightly fitting stopper or cork.

(2) Bleaching powder.

(3) A teaspoon.

(4) One litre of clear water.

Preparing a "stock solution"

Put three teaspoonsful of bleaching powder in the bottle.

Add clear water to the bottle until it is about half to three-quarters full.

Put the stopper on the bottle and shake it until any lumps of bleaching powder are broken up.

Fill the bottle to the top with clear water and shake the bottle a few times to mix the contents.

Note. This stock solution will look cloudy at first but after a while a white powder will settle at the bottom of the bottle. This does not matter because the white powder does not contain any disinfectant.

Store the stock solution in a dark place away from sunlight.

Disinfecting drinking water

If the water to be disinfected is clear and colourless, add one teaspoonful of the stock solution to each 10 litres of water (1.5 mg of Cl_2 per litre).

If the drinking water is cloudy or coloured or muddy-looking, use two teaspoonsful of stock solution for each 10 litres of drinking water (3 mg of Cl_2 per litre).

After adding the stock solution stir the water with a clean stick.

Then let it stand for 30 minutes to allow the chlorine enough time to disinfect the water.

9. Other techniques described in this book

Anatomical diagrams

The purpose of these diagrams is to help the trainers of community health workers in their teaching.

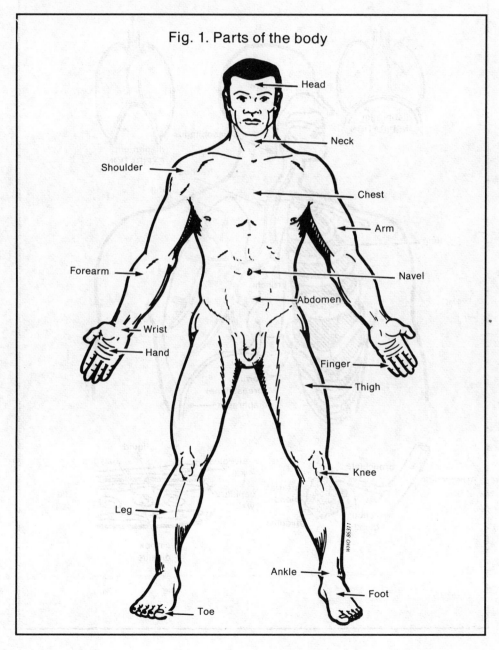

Fig. 1. Parts of the body

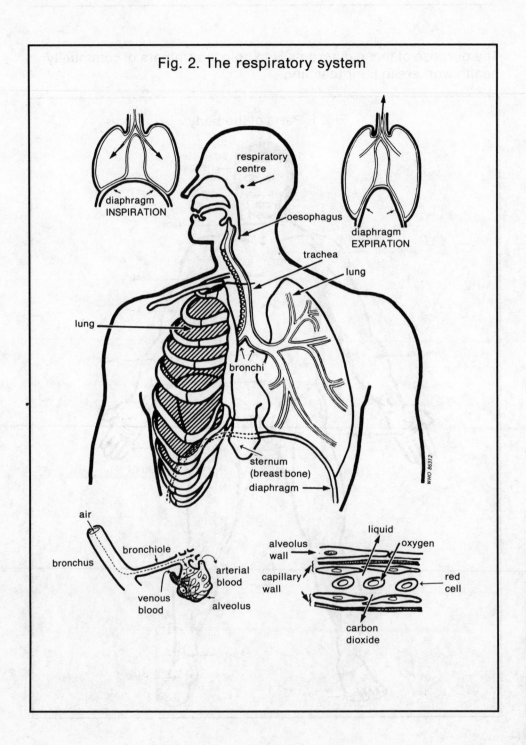

Fig. 2. The respiratory system

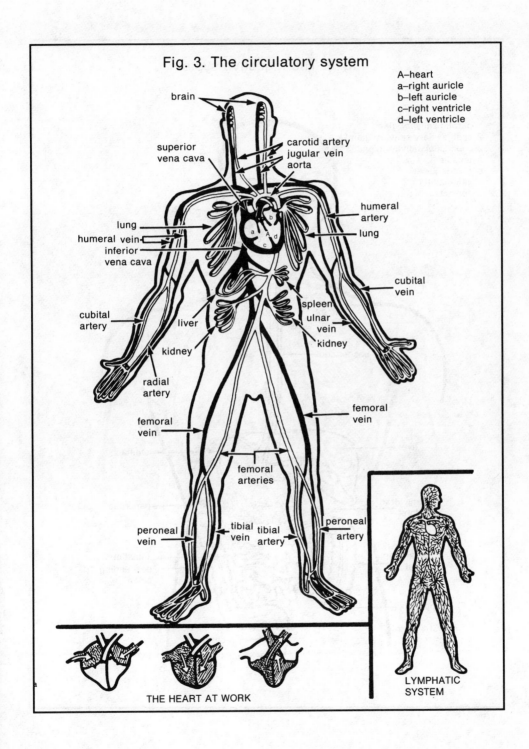

Fig. 3. The circulatory system

A–heart
a–right auricle
b–left auricle
c–right ventricle
d–left ventricle

brain

superior
vena cava

carotid artery
jugular vein
aorta

humeral
artery

lung
humeral vein
inferior
vena cava

lung

cubital
vein

cubital
artery

liver

kidney

spleen
ulnar
vein

kidney

radial
artery

femoral
vein

femoral
vein

femoral
arteries

peroneal
vein

tibial
vein

tibial
artery

peroneal
artery

THE HEART AT WORK

LYMPHATIC
SYSTEM

409

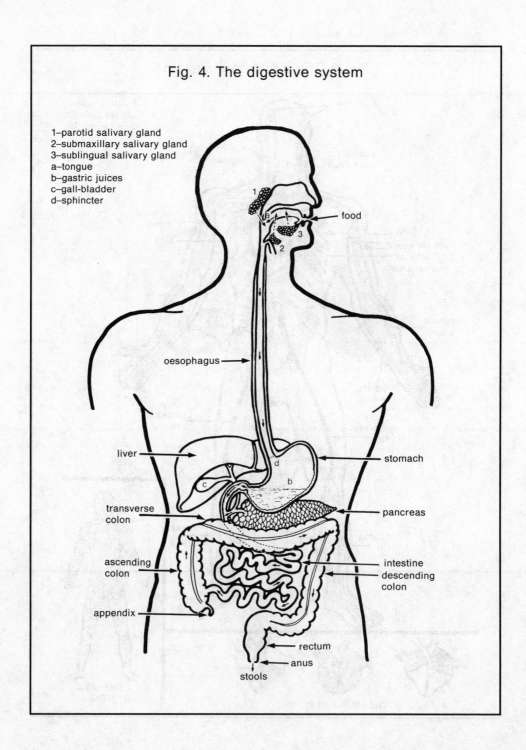

Fig. 4. The digestive system

1–parotid salivary gland
2–submaxillary salivary gland
3–sublingual salivary gland
a–tongue
b–gastric juices
c–gall-bladder
d–sphincter

food

oesophagus

liver

stomach

transverse
colon

pancreas

ascending
colon

intestine

descending
colon

appendix

rectum

anus

stools

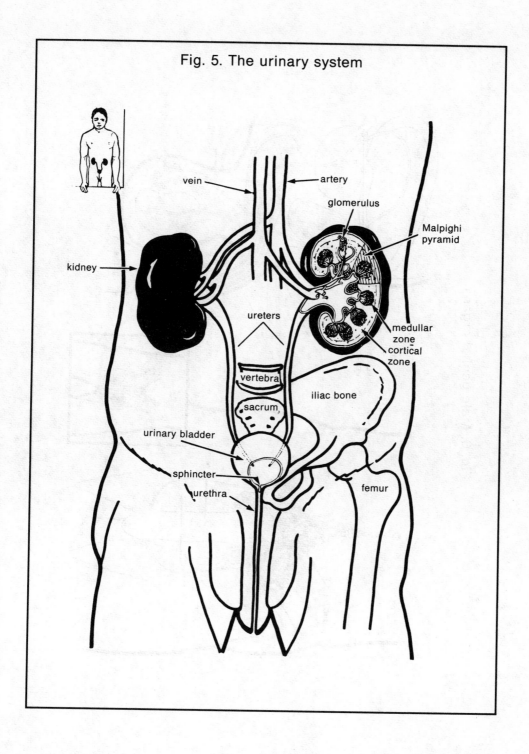

Fig. 5. The urinary system

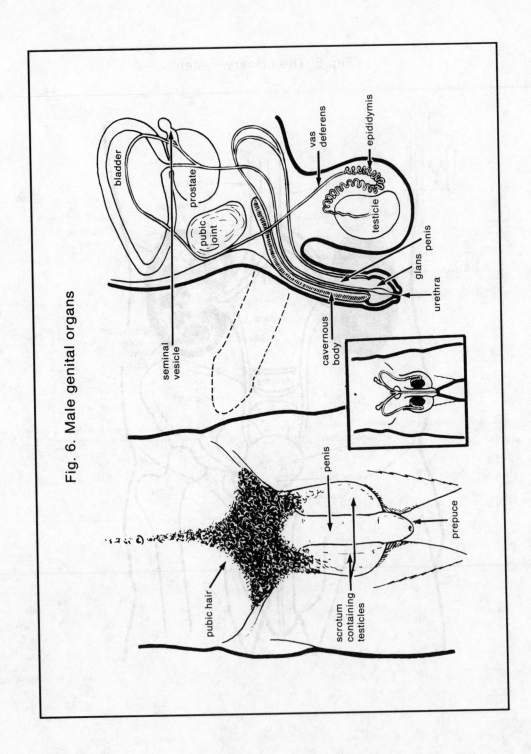

Fig. 6. Male genital organs

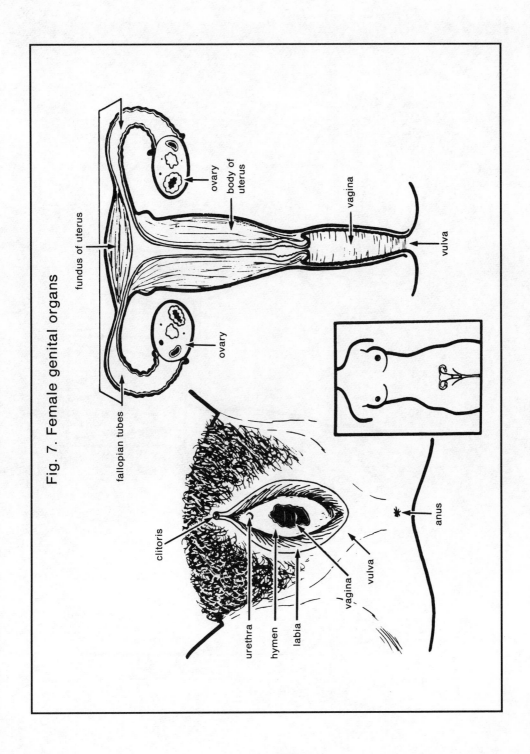

Fig. 7. Female genital organs

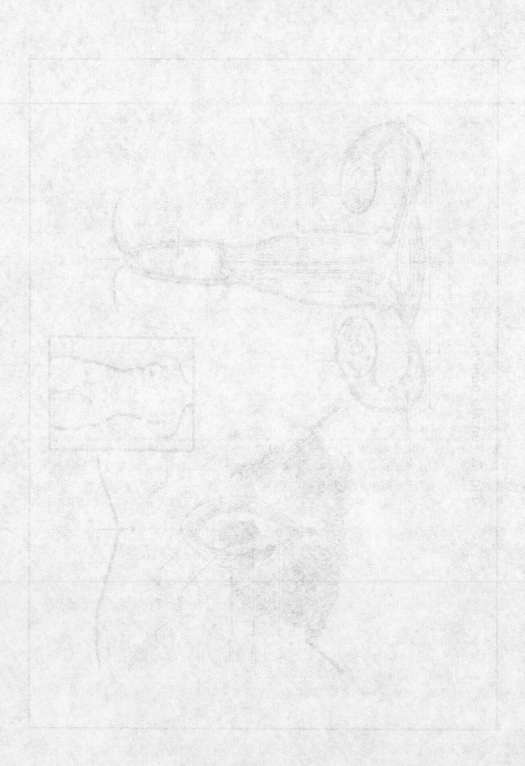

Explanation of terms and index

A

abscess: a lump of pus (page 311)

abdomen: *see* belly

abdominal: of the belly

accidents: *see under*: bites, burns, fracture, poisoning, wounds.

activated charcoal: *see* charcoal, activated

afterbirth (placenta): a piece of flesh in the womb to which the cord is attached and which comes out of a woman shortly after she has had a baby (pages 129, 138)

aluminium hydroxide: a medicine used to ease belly pains (page 38)

anaemia: a weakness of the blood, often due to bleeding or lack of iron in the diet (pages 298, 303)

aspirin: medicine that reduces pain and fever (page 381)

B

bacitracin: *see* neomycin/bacitracin ointment

BCG: the name of the vaccine against tuberculosis (TB); the initials stand for Bacille Calmette-Guérin (page 83)

bandage: a strip of cloth, which is wrapped around a part of the body when there is a wound or a broken bone (pages 392–396)

belly (abdomen), **belly pains** (page 230)

benzoic + salicylic acid: a medicine used for treating scabies (itch) (page 381)

benzyl benzoate: a medicine used for treating skin diseases (fungi) (page 381)

bilharziasis: *see* schistosomiasis

bites (page 266)

bleaching powder: a chemical used for disinfecting (cleaning) water (page 403)

bleeding: flow of blood (page 256)

blister: a lump on the skin filled with watery liquid (page 244)

boil: to heat water to 100 °C

boil: inflamed lump on the skin with pus, caused by germs (page 311)

bowel movement: passing of stools

breast-feeding (pages 156, 186)
burns (page 242)

C

C: Celsius (e.g., 37 °C)
cataract: an eye disease of old people leading to loss of sight (giving the impression of seeing through a cloud) (pages 94, 290)
charcoal, activated: a medicine used against diarrhoea (page 381)
chickenpox: a usually mild disease of children, which produces raised spots or small blisters on the skin (page 278)
childbirth: birth of a baby (page 127)
chlorination: the mixing of chlorine (bleaching powder) with water to disinfect (page 403)
chlorine: *see* bleaching powder
chloroquine: a medicine used against malaria (page 381)
chronic illness: an illness of a long duration (page 88)
CHW: community health worker
coil: a kind of intrauterine device (page 162)
colostrum: first milk that comes out from the breast after delivery of a baby (page 129)
committee: a group of persons appointed for a special function (e.g. community committee)
communicable disease: disease that spreads easily from one person to another (e.g., measles, tuberculosis)
community: people living in the same locality (the public)
community development: social activity in which members of a community meet to discuss their common needs and plan action to improve the living conditions of the whole community
competence: ability required to carry out a task
compress: a clean cloth used for dressing a wound (page 312)
condom: an elastic sheath worn on the penis during sexual intercourse to prevent pregnancy (page 161)
constipation: difficulty in defecating or the passing of hard stools
consultation: visit by a patient to get advice
contraceptive: a means of preventing pregnancy (page 159)
convulsions: violent involuntary movements (page 331)

cord: umbilical cord; cord that joins a baby to its mother (pages 129, 137, 139)

cure: to restore to health; recovery from an illness

D

defecate: to pass stools (*see* stool), to have a bowel movement

dehydration: the state of someone who has lost a lot of water from his body (e.g. during diarrhoea) (page 218)

delivery: giving birth (page 127)

dengue: an infectious disease transmitted by mosquitos, causing fever, rash and acute pains in the joints (page 71)

diaphragm: a circular contraceptive made of thin rubber which is put over the opening of the womb (cervix) to prevent pregnancy (page 162)

diarrhoea: passing of at least three liquid stools a day (page 217)

diphtheria: a usually severe infectious disease of the throat in which the inside of the throat becomes white (page 190)

disabled people: people who have something wrong with their body or brain; handicapped persons (page 97)

discharge: a yellowish or whitish liquid that comes out of, for example, the nose, the ear, the eye, the penis, the vagina

disinfect: to clean; to kill germs

dracunculosis: an infection of the skin caused by guinea worms (page 74)

dress: to clean a wound or burn and put a bandage on it

dressing: a clean strip of cloth used to cover a wound or burn

E

egg: a tiny cell produced inside the mother, which joins the father's sperm to produce a baby

epidemic: when several people catch the same disease at about the same time (page 25)

epilepsy: a disease of the brain which causes unconsciousness and convulsions (fits) (page 328)

ergometrine: a medicine used to stop bleeding after delivery or miscarriage (page 381)

excreta: stools
excreta, disposal of (page 59)
eye diseases (page 285)

F

faeces: stools
family planning: using contraceptive methods (condom, coil, etc.) to limit the number of children to that desired by the family (page 158)
fertilizer: a substance or product that makes plants grow faster and better (page 58)
fever: body temperature higher than 37.5°C (page 207)
feverish: said of a patient who is not well and whose temperature is over 37.5°C
filariasis: a disease, caused by a small worm and transmitted by certain flies and mosquitos, which may lead to great swelling of the legs, blindness, or infections of the skin (page 71)
fit: convulsions (page 328)
fluke: a small worm (carried by snails) that causes schistosomiasis (page 325)
fluoride: a chemical that is mixed with water or toothpaste to keep the teeth healthy (page 305)
flush (hot): a redness of the face with a feeling of heat
fodder: dried grass, straw, hay, etc. for feeding cattle
food safety (page 46)
forceps: a special instrument for holding objects; surgical pincers
FP: family planning
fracture: a broken bone (page 260)
fungus (plural fungi): a tiny plant that may grow on the skin and cause disease (page 278)

G

genital: of the sex organs
genitals: sex organs (pages 412, 413)

gentian violet: a liquid that is put on the skin to clean wounds and prevent infections (page 381)

germs: very small living animals that attack the human body (they can be seen only with a powerful microscope)

growth chart: a chart for recording the weight of a growing child at regular intervals (page 177)

H

haemorrhage: bleeding

handicapped person: a person suffering from a mental or physical disability, e.g., a person who cannot use his arms, hands, or legs in a normal way, or a person who cannot learn like other people (see also disabled people) (page 98)

headache: pain in the head (page 225)

high blood pressure: a condition related to the heart in which the patient may have a severe headache with or without a feeling of giddiness (page 228)

hookworm: a blood-sucking small worm that causes a disease in the intestines (page 298)

home visiting: (page 333)

housing (page 29)

hygiene: cleanliness, healthy habits (page 77)

I

immunization: making people resistant to disease by giving a vaccine (page 190)

impetigo: an infection of the skin with discharge of pus; can be passed from one person to another (page 278)

incision: cut (often made with a blade)

infection: entry of a germ into the body through the mouth or skin producing fever, pain, diarrhoea, coughing, redness, or pus or other discharge

injection: liquid (medicine) put into the body (usually the buttock or the arm) using a needle and syringe (page 388)

intestinal worms: worms that cause disease in the belly (intestines) (page 294)

intrauterine device (IUD): a loop, ring-, or coil-shaped contraceptive put into the womb to prevent pregnancy (page 162)

iodine (tincture): a liquid that is put on skin for cleaning wounds (page 381)

ipecacuanha: a medicine used to cause vomiting (page 381)

iron sulfate: a medicine used to cure weakness caused by a lot of bleeding or certain kinds of malnutrition (page 381)

IUD: intrauterine device

J

jaundice: yellowness of the skin, eyes, and tissues, and dark yellow urine

joint: the part of the body where two bones meet, e.g., the knee or the ankle (page 234)

L

labour: the process of giving birth (page 127)

latrine: an enclosed place for passing stools and urinating (*see* excreta, disposal of) (page 59)

learning objective: what a community health worker should know or be able to do after he has studied a problem or practised a skill and which he did not know or could not do before

leprosy: a chronic infectious disease of the skin which causes disfigurement of the affected parts (page 282)

living standards (standard of living): level of material comfort (housing, food, clothing, education, occupation, etc.) available to a person or community

loop: a type of intrauterine device (page 162)

lumps: a swelling on the body that may or may not be hard (page 310)

M

malaria: a disease causing high fever and shivering (passed on by mosquitos) (page 209)

malnutrition: a condition resulting from being underfed or fed with the wrong foods (page 183)

maternal care: care of mothers

measles: an infectious disease of children causing red spots on the skin, red eyes, and fever (transmitted mainly by coughing) (pages 190, 278)

mebendazole: a medicine used against intestinal worms (roundworms and pinworms) (page 381)

medicines: drugs used for curing diseases (page 379)

mental health (page 315)

mental disorders: diseases of the mind (page 315)

metronidazole: a medicine used for the treatment of trichomoniasis (page 381)

microscope: an instrument used for seeing germs and other very tiny objects that cannot be seen normally

migraine: a long-lasting headache with a feeling of sickness (page 226)

milestones: marks that indicate progress, e.g., when a small child starts walking without help

milestones of development: an event in the progress of development (page 182)

ml: millilitre (1000 ml = 1 litre)

mouth, diseases of (page 304)

mouth-to-mouth resuscitation: a way of reviving someone whose breathing has stopped (page 397)

mucus: a thick slimy liquid produced inside the body

N

nasal: of the nose

nausea: feeling of sickness which comes before vomiting

navel: the place where the cord is attached at birth (page 152)

neomycin/bacitracin ointment: a medicine used for treating infections of the skin (page 381)

niclosamide: a medicine used against intestinal worms (flatworms and tapeworms (page 381)

nutrition (page 175)

O

ocular: of the eye

ointment: any oily or paste-like medicine for putting on the skin (or in some cases for putting in the eyes)

old people, care of (page 93)

ophthalmic: of the eye

oral rehydration salts: a packet of powder to dissolve in drinking-water for making oral rehydration fluid for treating diarrhoea and dehydration (pages 221, 381)

ORS: oral rehydration salts

P

pain, in the belly: *see* belly pains

pain, in the head: *see* headache

pains in the joints (page 234)

pap: semi-liquid mashed food for infants (page 188)

penicillin: a medicine used against infectious diseases (page 382)

penis: the male sex organ (page 412)

period: loss of blood from the vagina, which occurs every month in women who are not pregnant, between the ages of about 15 and 44 years (page 103)

PHC: primary health care

phenobarbital: a medicine used to calm excited persons and to help them to sleep; also used to treat people who have epilepsy (page 382)

pill: any medicine shaped like a tiny ball; contraceptive pills are medicines taken by mouth to prevent pregnancy (page 161)

piperazine: a medicine against roundworms and small worms (page 382)

placenta: *see* afterbirth

poisoning: effects of accidental or deliberate intake of something poisonous (page 273)

poliomyelitis (polio): an infectious disease that may cause paralysis (page 190)

postnatal care: care of a baby and the mother after birth (page 146)

pregnancy: when a woman is expecting a baby (page 101)
pregnant woman: a woman who is expecting a baby
premature: word used to describe a child who is born early and who has a weight of less than 2500 grams (page 153)
procaine benzylpenicillin: a kind of penicillin, *see* penicillin (page 382)
prostate: a gland in men located under the urinary bladder; in elderly men it may swell and cause difficulties in urinating (page 97)
purgative: a medicine taken to make it easier to pass stools
pulse: heart beats felt at the wrist (page 397)
pus: a yellowish liquid that comes out of an infected wound or boil (pages 254, 312)

R

rabies: a disease, mainly of dogs, foxes, or bats, which can be passed on to humans through bites of those animals (page 266)
records: information written down for future use (page 362)
refer: send to the nearest hospital or health centre (page 354)
refuse: rubbish, dirt, or waste material that is thrown away (page 54)
rehydration: replacement of the water lost from the body when dehydration occurs (especially in diarrhoea) (page 219)
reports (page 369)
respiratory diseases: diseases of the lungs (*see* cough (page 211) and tuberculosis (page 82))
retinol (vitamin A): a medicine used for the treatment of certain eye diseases (page 382)
ringworm: a skin disease (caused by certain fungi) that produces round red itchy patches on the body (page 281)
rubbish: refuse, dirt, or waste material that is thrown away (page 54)
runny nose: flowing of watery mucus from the nose

S

scab: a small piece of hard dry skin

scabies: an infectious skin disease that is easily passed on to other people and which causes intense itching (page 279)

schistosomiasis: a disease causing blood in the urine or in the faeces; it is caused by a small worm that lives in water-snails and enters the body through the skin (pages 74, 325)

schoolchildren (page 65)

sexual intercourse: sexual relations between a man and woman

sexually transmitted diseases: diseases that are passed on during sexual intercourse (page 320)

sheath: *see* condom

silver nitrate: a medicine used to prevent eye diseases in newborn babies (page 382)

shock (page 256)

skin diseases (page 277)

skinfold: a crease in the skin

sperm: the fluid produced by the man during sexual intercourse; it contains tiny cells that join with the woman's egg to produce a baby (page 103)

splint: a piece of wood or other material used to support a broken leg or arm (page 262)

sputum: mucus coughed up by a person (page 213)

sticking plaster: a clean cloth that is sticky and is used to hold dressings in place and to close wounds (page 252)

stiff: rigid, not flexible (stiff neck, page 227)

stillbirth: birth of a dead child

stool: what the body passes out through the anus; faeces

stretcher: a bed that can be carried by two people to transport a sick person (page 399)

sulfamethoxazole + trimethoprim: a medicine used to treat infections (page 382)

sunken eyes: a sign of dehydration (page 218)

swelling: enlargement of a limb or of part of a limb; may also be a small lump

syphilis: a disease transmitted by sexual contact that causes a sore on the genitals followed by red spots, and later on, various severe complaints affecting blood vessels, nerves, the brain, etc. (page 323)

syringe: an instrument for giving injections (page 388)

T

tablet: a flat, round pill of medicine
task: a specific piece of work
TB: tuberculosis (page 82)
TBA: traditional birth attendant (page 101)
techniques: ways of doing things
teeth, diseases of (page 306)
temperature: internal heat of the body; can be measured with
   thermometer (37 °C = normal temperature, above
   37.5 °C = fever, above 39 °C = high fever) (page 385)
tetanus: an infectious disease that causes severe muscular
   contractions; often affects newborn babies if dirt is applied to the
   umbilical cord; adults may get this disease if they leave their
   wounds untreated (pages 154, 190)
tetanus antitoxin serum (ATS): a medicine used to prevent and treat
   tetanus (page 382)
tetracycline: a medicine used against certain infections (page 382)
tiredness (page 300)
traditional birth attendant (page 101)
trichomoniasis: a mild venereal disease producing vaginal
   discharge and itching and sometimes causing a burning feeling
   when urinating (page 320)
tuberculosis: a chronic disease, mostly of the lungs, that is easily
   passed on from person to person (page 82)

U

ulcer: an open sore
umbilical cord: *see* cord
uterus: *see* womb

V

vaccination: *see* immunization
vaccine: a medicine (made from the germs that cause a disease)
   that gives the body resistance against the disease (page 190)
vagina: the birth canal (*see* female genitals in Annex 3) (page
   413)

vectors of disease: animals or insects that pass the germs of diseases to human beings (page 70)

vegetable oil: oil that comes from plants

venereal diseases *see* sexually transmitted diseases

vitamin: a substance present in many foodstuffs (fruit, butter, oil, milk, etc.) which is essential for the normal growth and nutrition of man, e.g., vitamin A is found mainly in oil, milk, butter, fruit, and carrots, and is essential for good sight (*see* retinol)

vomiting (pages 110, 275)

vulva: the opening of the vagina (external genitals of females) (*see* Annex 3) (page 413)

W

water supply (page 36)

weakness: (page 300) *see also* anaemia

whooping cough (pertussis): an infectious disease of children which causes a short violent cough followed by long noisy intake of breath, and sometimes by vomiting (page 190)

womb: the pouch in which a baby grows inside the mother (pages 108, 130, 413)

women's health problems (page 167)

worms: parasites (small animals) that live in the body (e.g., in the belly (intestines) or on the skin) and cause disease (page 294)

wounds (page 247)

Y

yaws: a skin disease that occurs mainly in tropical countries and which produces red sores; if left untreated it causes joint pains and other problems (page 282)

yellow fever: a severe tropical disease, passed on by mosquitos, causing high fever and jaundice (page 71)

Part 2

Guidelines for training community health workers

Guidelines for training community health workers [1]

1. Creating conditions for learning

What the teacher must do

Before training begins, the teacher should learn about the students: who they are, where they come from, what has been their previous experience at school or at work. He should discover by means of standard tests what each student can already do, e.g., the level of reading and writing ability, or what each student already knows about health care. This will help the teacher to adjust the teaching according to the students' previous knowledge and ability and their capacity to learn.

There may be minimum requirements or qualifications that students need in order to join the programme (e.g., primary school education, ability to read and write the local language, minimum age). Encouraging students to talk about their own backgrounds is another way of finding out more about them. At the same time, the students can share and compare their experiences, and from this the teacher can learn what the students expect from the training programme. This period of adjustment—the orientation period— may last for a few days or longer.

Next, the teacher has four basic tasks. First, he must know very well the tasks for which the students are to be trained and must make clear to the students exactly what they have to learn to do. In this book, the list of learning objectives at the beginning of each unit states exactly what the student should be able to do after studying that unit. The health authority and the teachers may set up other learning objectives, if there are other problems and tasks for which community health workers need to be trained.

---

[1] See also: Guilbert, J.-J. *Educational handbook for health personnel*. Second revised edition. Geneva, World Health Organization, 1987 (WHO Offset Publication, No. 35); and Abbatt, F. R. *Teaching for better learning*. Geneva, World Health Organization, 1980.

Second, the teacher must decide exactly how he will find out whether the students have learned to perform these tasks. This is usually done through tests at the end of each unit and of the entire period of training in which the performance of the students is assessed. As a rule, the best way of testing is to watch the students while they are doing the tasks and check against a list prepared by the teacher before the training begins.

Third, the teacher must set up the conditions in which the student will be able to practise the required task until he can do it properly; the conditions should be similar to those in which he will later work. For each of the learning objectives given at the beginning of each unit the teacher should arrange a training exercise, or a number of different exercises, to enable the student to learn to do what the objective describes. For most skills or groups of skills the student must be given repeated opportunities to practise until he can perform the task adequately.

Fourth, the teacher checks the student's performance of the task against the check-list he has prepared earlier and decides whether the student has reached an acceptable level of performance. If the student fails in one or more parts, the teacher should explain to him why he has failed and should provide more opportunity for the student to practise those parts of the task.

After some experience with each unit, the teacher should be able to tell whether any of the objectives need to be changed or omitted, whether new objectives are necessary, whether the conditions provided for the students to learn to perform the tasks need to be improved, and whether the tests used to assess the students' performance are adequate. In this way the training programme can be improved.

The conditions for learning

It should be noted that the learning objectives of each unit begin with the sentence 'After studying this unit you should be able to . . .'. The emphasis is therefore on ability to do something, to perform tasks. It is not so much on knowledge or memory. Some of the tasks to be learned are simple and some are very complex.

Students can learn tasks only by practising them repeatedly under supervision, until they have reached a level of performance that is acceptable according to agreed standards. The teacher must be skilled in methods that permit students to "learn by doing". One of the functions of the teacher and the institution or organization that provides training is to provide the conditions in which all the students can practise the required tasks under supervision until they have mastered them.

Other methods will often be necessary, for instance, in teaching the principles of health care or providing information needed by the trainees to be able to perform the tasks. However, the training course, whether short or long, must be for the greatest part a practical course in which students do practical exercises, which gradually become more complex.

Practical training of this kind needs practice settings such as health centres, communities, and families where students can practise the necessary tasks under supervision. However, it is not always possible or necessary, or even advisable, to provide a real health-centre setting for training, especially before a student has mastered basic skills. For example, a teacher will not allow a student to use a real patient or any person when learning to give an injection. Instead he will probably arrange for the student to practise on an object such as an orange or a rubber ball. Students can practise on one another, for example, in learning how to count the pulse, take the temperature, put on a bandage, or ask questions about health problems. Thus, classrooms or laboratories are also needed, where students can learn before they begin work with patients and their families. For this kind of training, students must be organized in groups small enough to permit every student to practise the tasks expected of him.

As well as providing conditions in which the students can learn to perform properly the tasks they are assigned, a good teacher always ensures that the conditions are such that he can assess fully and fairly the students' ability to do correctly what they are expected to do. Asking students to explain orally or in writing how to make a filter for water or how to deliver a baby is not the best way of judging their ability to do these tasks.

From simple to more complex tasks

As a general rule students should learn simple tasks before learning more complex ones. Complex health care tasks at the community level are made up of several simple tasks. A good teacher can break complex tasks down into their simple components, and then help students to put them together into complex tasks again.

An example of a simple task is boiling a litre of water. An example of a less simple task is making correctly an oral rehydration solution. A more complex task is giving a drink of this mixture to a dehydrated baby. Another kind of complex task is working well in a health team.

While it will take a short time for the students to learn simple tasks, complex tasks will take a long time. Many of the complex tasks will be fully learned only by actual working experience after the student leaves the training course. Sometimes the students may need to come back several times for more training before acquiring the ability to do a complex task completely and efficiently.

The ability to do tasks fades away if the tasks are not performed fairly regularly. Therefore, when community health workers return to the training school to learn new tasks, the opportunity should be taken to give them refresher training for tasks learned previously. It is much easier and it takes much less time to relearn tasks that have been learned well once but not used for a long time.

In general, students should not be required to learn everything in this book in a single period of training. The training system should as far as possible permit the trainees to alternate periods of practice in the community and in health posts with periods of training and retraining at a training centre.

An example of a complex task: ability to work in a health team

A person can almost always do something for himself (or a mother can do something for her child) when faced with a problem. The CHW may be able to teach people to do some more things for themselves. But the CHW can do only what he is trained to do, and if he cannot solve a problem he must seek the help of others who know what to do. If the problem is an illness, he may seek the help of a nurse or medical assistant; if some families have too little food after a poor harvest, the CHW may need to consult the village council, a community development officer, or an agricultural officer; if the problem is a dirty well, the health inspector or sanitarian may need to be called in. This way of working with others is called *teamwork*. Teamwork is necessary because health problems are of many types, and people who are specialists in different fields can solve different problems. To do his share, the CHW must understand how the work of these other community workers can improve the health of the people and how to work together with them in the best way. Learning to work in a team is like learning any other task. The CHW can learn teamwork tasks only by practising them by working in actual teams. The teachers can help the trainees by discussing with them their own experiences of working in teams. Thus, during training the teacher must arrange for students to see how health teams work and provide opportunities for students to perform tasks that require teamwork, both in health-care teams and in multidisciplinary teams, comprising, for example, health workers, schoolteachers, agricultural workers, and community development workers. The teacher should also make a special effort to arrange for a part of the training to be carried out in the actual teams in which the students will later work.

Developing students' learning abilities

It is a function of the teacher to help the students to become "self-learners", i.e., to learn by themselves independently of a teacher, from this and other books, and from experience. Therefore, the teacher must make sure that each student can *read and write* at least to the level required for working from this book. The students' reading and writing skills may therefore need to be tested at or before the beginning of training, and the student must be helped to deal with any weaknesses in reading and writing that are discovered.

In this regard, the teacher should pay particular attention to familiarizing students with the style of this book. This is because although the writing style is very simple, many students may not be used to it. Many sentences in this book begin with a common root and continue with many branches. For example:

"The tasks of a teacher are: *the common root*

■ to be available to students when they need him

■ to define learning objectives properly

■ to prepare learning aids *the branches*

■ to assess students' work

■ to supervise students' progress

■ to set an example, etc."

The purpose of this approach was to avoid writing many long sentences. The teachers will find that once the students get used to this style, they will find this book very easy to use.

Apart from being able to read and write, the students must also be *numerate*. This means that they should be able to use numbers in their work, e.g., for making calculations, keeping records of simple statistics, and making charts. Thus, the teacher must make sure that the students know basic arithmetic well enough to do their work and to continue to learn by themselves. Similarly, they must be trained to interpret and use numbers correctly, to make simple calculations, and to use simple statistics, such as rates.

The teacher must never take for granted that the students are adequately literate and numerate, and should never reject or fail them if they are later found not be so without giving them a chance to improve.

The students must be physically and intellectually able to perform the tasks for which they are to be trained. They must be willing to learn and perform the tasks well. They must be in good health so that they can be good students and health workers and so that they do not pass on diseases to other students or to the people in the community.

Students should have good *habits of study* and methods of study. One way in which the teacher can help students to become good learners is to make them responsible for large parts of their own learning. The teacher should show them how to check their own progress and how to use the resources of the training centre (books, equipment, other students, teachers, supervisors, health workers) when they need help or have difficulties in learning. In the case of students who are naturally inclined to act independently, the teachers should encourage them to be independent in learning by giving them a certain amount of freedom especially in performing tasks. Other students may be passive and inclined to expect the teacher to tell them everything because this is how they were taught at school. The teacher must at all times resist this. He should stimulate students to act independently and reward them for doing so. They must not be discouraged by mistakes; people learn from mistakes.

The teacher must remember that learning is a personal process and that individuals have their own distinct learning styles.

Other skills that students need to learn in order to work with people are *social skills*, i.e., the ability to relate easily, but respectfully and firmly, with most people—individuals and families, community leaders and other workers in the health services. In learning social skills the CHW must develop the ability to listen attentively to people, to encourage them to say what they want and to overcome shyness or guilt about a personal health problem. Students must be able to distinguish between what is important and what is not, and to remember the important parts of what people say.

The teacher should get to know the students individually by observing their behaviour when they are working in groups and by means of individual interviews. In every training exercise in which there is interaction between students and other people (e.g., other students in group discussions, patients and other family members, or other health workers) it is an important task of the teacher or the supervisor to observe the ways in which each student reacts and communicates and to provide opportunities for more practise to those students who have difficulty in communicating. A special part of the teacher's day should be set aside for individual interviews with students for this purpose.

Students who are weak in social skills may benefit from special attention, especially if they lack confidence in relating to other people. They may need a very gradual exposure to situations that cause them anxiety and stress. The teacher will need to protect them from too much stress in the early stages of training and to encourage them by showing them the progress they make in social skills. At the same time the teacher should watch out for the student who seems to be too confident, who may make relationships too easily, but who may not be sincere. Both types of student may have difficulties in learning the basic social skills needed in their work.

Sometimes it happens that a student has so much difficulty in working with other people (e.g., because the person is too aggressive or too withdrawn) that teachers and supervisors may decide that he or she should not be assigned to community health work. Sometimes such students can be trained for other health tasks, e.g., laboratory or mechanical work.

2. Evaluating the performance of students

1. How to know whether the purposes of training have been attained

To evaluate the performance of students is to measure the level of performance and judge whether the students can do what they have been trained to do. Evaluation is an essential part of training.

Evaluation should consider not only the individual student's performance, but also the training programme itself. It is obvious that, if the training programme is defective in one or more respects, the product (the student's performance) will also be unsatisfactory. Therefore, in education and training we should use both kinds of evaluation: the student's performance and the effectiveness of the training programme.

Teachers must evaluate the performance of the students, and the students need to be able to evaluate their own performance, in order to discover:

- how well the students are learning what they should be learning
- why they are not doing better
- in which areas they are strong or weak
- how they can be helped to improve their learning
- in what ways the training programme needs to be improved.

Such evaluation is a very important way of helping students to learn. It can encourage students who are doing well to continue to do well and to do even better. It not only shows the areas in which the students need to improve their performance, but also the areas of the programme itself (including the teaching) that need to be modified.

Students should take part in evaluating their own performance. They must be told the results of this evaluation so that they become aware of their weaknesses and strengths and can build on the strengths. Evaluation during training, when done properly, is intended to help students to learn, and to show in what respects they need to improve; it should not be a basis for punishment.

For teachers, the evaluation of students, based on properly constructed performance assessment tests, is the best way to learn about the quality of their own teaching. Teachers should facilitate the students' efforts to learn. Often, students do not or cannot learn because the teacher pays no attention to their weak points or strong points and thus gives no encouragement. This is not good teaching.

We can judge whether a programme is good or not by testing the extent to which it results in the students being able to perform the tasks expected of them at the end of the training. Also, we can discover which parts of the training programme need to be improved, dropped, or replaced. We can do this by examining the students during and at the end of the course, and also by getting information about the quality of their work when they are employed in the community. For example, if many children are getting diarrhoea in different communities it may mean that the community health workers are not doing their work properly, and that training needs to be improved or continued in the community after the students have finished the course.

2. When should student performance be evaluated?

Evaluation should go on all the time. It should be possible to judge continuously the value of the learning objectives of a course so that they may be revised if necessary. There are ways of evaluating every element of an educational programme: students, teachers, teaching exercises, learning aids, examination questions, performance check-lists, etc. Students should be evaluated during the process of learning so that teachers can see how they are progressing and where they need further help or individual attention. Later, when they work in the community, there are ways of evaluating the training programme by finding out (1) whether what they learned is appropriate to their work; (2) whether there are any problems or tasks for which they have not been adequately trained; (3) whether the CHWs are working with interest and satisfaction; (4) whether they are staying in their work; and (5) whether the community is satisfied with the services they give. This information is then given to those who plan and carry out the training programme so that they can make any changes that may be indicated. Whenever an element of a programme is evaluated, the information obtained should be used to improve the programme.

A good educational system continues to support its students even after they have begun to work in the health service or for a community. This is so because there are always more skills to be learnt. Also, CHWs will need to improve the skills they already have. Their supervisors, for instance, can identify the parts of their performance in which they may be weak and either help them to improve or arrange further training for them. The evaluation of the performance of CHWs in the community will show what continuing education support is needed.

3. How to evaluate performance

Evaluation should form an important part of all learning and teaching activities. Since the training of CHWs is concerned mainly with the students' ability to perform practical tasks, all tests should measure this ability. The teacher or supervisor should have a check-list of skills that the student must demonstrate in performing the tasks (in a group or individually). The teacher or supervisor then observes the student doing the task (e.g., making a filter for water) and checks against the check-list how well he performs the important parts of it. At the same time, or afterwards, the teacher or supervisor can ask questions to test the student's understanding of why he did certain things and the reasons why he did not do certain others. The usual kinds of paper or oral examinations are *not* suitable for testing students' ability to perform most health-care tasks.

4. The qualities of a good test

Four things are important for the teacher to remember when testing the performance of students during and at the end of a training course:

(1) All tests must be *valid*. This means that a test must measure what it sets out to measure. A test that only requires the student to recall or repeat what a teacher said, or what is written in a book, is a test of memory; such a test should be used only if the teacher wants to test a student's ability to remember or recall something. To test the student's ability to perform a task, the examiner must set up a performance test. In order to test an intellectual skill, e.g.,

to solve a problem for which the student must reason and make decisions, the test must require the student to use the necessary intellectual skills.

(2) The test must also be *relevant*. It must measure the knowledge, skills, attitudes and behaviour it sets out to measure. If the teacher wants to find out how much the student knows and what he can do about a problem (e.g., burns), he must ask the student only those questions and observe only those actions that are relevant to burns.

(3) The test must be *reliable*. It should give the expected results (the same answers and the same performance) in most cases. If there are a number of different correct answers or responses to the same test, it is not a reliable test and should not be used.

(4) The test should be *objective*. This means that different independent examiners should be able to agree on what is the correct or a satisfactory response. If the teacher wants to avoid making a wrong judgement about a learning experience, he can prepare in advance the answers he will accept as correct for particular questions, as shown below:

Questions	*Answers*
When does a medicine become a poison?	■ When it is given to the wrong person.
	■ When the wrong amount is given.
When is a medicine useless?	■ When the patient does not take it.
	■ When it is not taken at the right time.
	■ When it is not taken for long enough.
Along with the medicine what information must you give to the patient so that he takes the medicine in the right way.	■ How much medicine he should take.
	■ How often he should take it.
	■ How long he should take it for.

5. Using properly the results of evaluation

In any evaluation, it will probably be found that the students fall into three groups:

(1) those who know but cannot do

(2) those who do not know but can do

(3) those who know and can do.

The aim of the training programme should be to produce CHWs of the third category—i.e., those who know and can do. Therefore, the teacher must compare the results of evaluation with the learning objectives to see whether all students know everything that they should know about the tasks and can perform the tasks in the way they should. If some students are found to be weak in one of the two areas, they should be helped to correct the weak points. For example, a student who does not know all that he should about a task but can perform the task, (e.g., he can very well weigh a baby but he does not understand the danger of the baby becoming thinner) must spend more time learning to understand this danger. In the case of a student who knows about a task and can answer questions and teach others well but cannot perform correctly the important tasks, such as applying a dressing or giving an injection, the teacher must spend more time on helping him learn practical work.

3. Examples of learning modules

Definition of a learning module

A "learning module" is a planned set of activities which assist the student (the CHW) in learning a particular group of skills.

Learning modules can be put together for each unit presented in the working guide (Part 1). They can make learning and teaching easier by presenting the topics in a logical way.

Following are two examples of learning modules based on two of the units in the book. These can be further expanded by the teacher.

- Child care and feeding (Unit 20)
- Burns (Unit 30)

The sequence is the following:

(1) State the problem.

(2) Define the learning objectives.

(3) Find out what the CHWs already know about the problem.

(4) Divide the learning content, as in the working guide, into what the trainees should know (knowledge) and what they should be able to do (skills).

(5) Build on what the trainees already know and can do.

(6) Select and list the learning and teaching methods in the order in which they best suit the learning objectives.

(7) Assess and evaluate the progress made by the CHWs.

The same process can be used for each of the topics dealt with in this book, as well as for others identified by the health authorities to meet the needs of a given community. Teacher-training centres and WHO, or other advisers, can assist you in this task, if necessary.

Example 1. Child care and feeding (Unit 20)

Learning objectives

After studying this unit, the trainee should be able to:

- Explain to parents why children should have regular health examinations during the first few years of life.

- Use the growth chart to discuss with parents a child's growth and what they can do to make sure that the child grows normally.

- Check the normal development of a child using the major milestones.

- Identify underfed children without using a growth chart.

- Advise mothers about foods that help children to grow and develop normally.

Finding out what the trainee already knows

Find out the answers to the following questions:

- What does the trainee think should be done to take good care of a child?

- Has he already seen or filled in a growth chart?

- Does he know at what age a baby normally walks, talks, has teeth, etc.?

- Has he already seen underfed children? How does he recognize them?

- Which foods does he think are good for children and which are bad?

Learning content

(1) The trainee *must know*:

- that the best way to check whether a child is eating enough or not is by watching his weight

- that weight is measured on a balance

- that weight should be recorded on a growth chart

- the four main milestones of development

- what foods should be given to children at different ages—less than 5 months, at 5 months, between 6 months and 1 year, and after 1 year

- which children need special attention.

(2) the trainee *must be able to*:

- weigh a child

- read a growth chart

- fill in a growth chart

- explain to the family of a child why it is important to fill in a growth chart

- advise the family what to do if a child is not growing well
- inform the supervisor about children that he cannot treat
- refer such children to the hospital or health centre
- report to the community committee.

Using what the trainee already knows

The previous knowledge of trainees will differ depending on their educational backgrounds. With regard to child care and feeding, they may be able to do the following:

- compare the ages and weights of healthy children with those of children who are not growing well
- explain what makes a baby grow and develop normally
- explain the local customs and habits about food and how to improve them
- explain the advantages of birth spacing
- feed children.

Learning/teaching methods

(1) *Observation of how mothers care for and feed their children.* The trainees can do this at the health clinic or at the homes of mothers. They could also find out about feeding practices in the community by talking to mothers.

(2) *Finding out what food is available in the community.* To do this, the trainees may be taken out on a trip to the market.

(3) *Talking with people about healthy nutrition.* Trainees could do this when they visit the market, or they may talk to people attending the health clinic.

(4) *Practising weighing children and recording weights on a growth chart.* The health clinic is the best place for doing this.

(5) *Group discussion.* The trainees could gather with other development workers and discuss problems of growing food for the growth and development needs of children.

Check-list for evaluation

There are two ways of evaluating trainees: by observation and by questioning.

(1) *By observation.* Observe the following:

- Before weighing the child did the trainee adjust the balance to the zero-level?
- Did he hold the child safely?
- Did he talk with the child or mother?
- Did he read the weight correctly?
- Did he write the weight correctly on the growth chart?

(2) *By questioning.* Ask the trainee the following questions:

- Is the weight of the child correct for his age?
- What would you advise the child's mother?
- How would you know whether the child is improving?
- What can you do to prevent the child from losing weight?

Example 2. Burns (Unit 30)

Learning objectives

After studying this unit, the trainee should be able to:

- Tell whether a burn covers a small or a large area of the skin.
- Tell when a patient with burns should be sent to the hospital or health centre.
- Decide what to do when a large area of the skin is burned.
- Take care of patients who only have a small area of the skin burned:
    - when they come less than 24 hours after the burn;
    - when they come more than 24 hours after the burn.
- Decide what to do in the case of chemical burns of the skin.

- Discuss with the community and suggest measures to prevent burns.

Finding out what the trainee already knows:

Has the trainee or a member of his family ever been burned?

How was the burn treated?

What happened to the person who was burned?

Learning content

(1) The trainee *must know*:

- how burns are caused
- how to prevent burns
- the dangers of a large area of skin being burned
- how to keep the burn clean and prevent infection
- what first aid to give to a person who has a large area of his skin burnt (how to take temperature, what medicines to give, how to give an injection, and the importance of giving fluids)
- how to recognize and treat patients who have only a small area of the skin burnt (how to recognize blisters and how to dress them)
- what advice to give to the family of the patient with burns
- how to recognize complications (fever, discharge, bad swelling) and when to refer the patient to hospital
- how to organize community gatherings for health education.

(2) The trainee *must be able to*:

- teach people how to prevent burns (protecting children from fire)
- give first aid
- give fluid
- take temperature
- give an injection of penicillin

- give other treatment
- send the patient to hospital
- follow up the patient's treatment
- refer in case of complication
- prepare and clean equipment.

Using what the trainee already knows

The knowledge of the trainees will differ depending on their educational background and how well they know the previous units. They may already know, for instance:

- how to dress a burn, give an injection, and take temperature
- how germs spread infection (described in the unit on fever)
- how flies increase the risk of infection (described in unit on getting rid of waste).

Learning/teaching methods

(1) *Observation of a patient with burns.* This will be best done in a health centre.

(2) *Practical experience in treating burns.* The trainee can practise giving treatment and dressing burns at the health centre.

(3) *Group discussion.* The trainees can discuss with the teacher the severe and mild complications of burns and how accidents involving burns happen and can be prevented.

(4) *Demonstration of dressing techniques.* The teacher can demonstrate to the students the different ways of dressing burns on different parts of the body.

Check-list for evaluation

There are two ways of evaluating trainees: by observation and by questioning.

(1) *By observation:* Observe the following:

- Did he wash his hands before dressing a burn?

- How did he examine the patient?
- Did he examine the patient gently?
- Did he speak with the patient and his family and reassure them?
- Did he give the right treatment? Was he able to judge rightly whether the burn was on a small or large area of the skin?
- Did he prepare the necessary equipment and clean it afterwards?
- Did he take the temperature and give the injection in the right way?
- Did he communicate with the community gathering in the right way when he told them about prevention of burns?

By questioning. Ask the following questions:

- When is a burn serious?
- Why is it important to give fluid to certain patients with burns?
- What complications can occur in a patient with burns?
- When should you send a patient with burns to the health centre or hospital?
- What are the various causes of burns?
- How can one prevent burns?
- How can the community help in preventing burns?

Part 3

Guidelines for adapting this book

Guidelines for adapting this book

1. Introduction

All those who work in the field and who are concerned with the training of community health workers (CHWs) know that the manuals and guides at their disposal are often ill-adapted to their needs. This is due to the fact that local conditions vary considerably from one country to another and even from one province to another.

Educators have often come to the conclusion that the best teaching/ learning material is that prepared on the spot taking local conditions into account as much as possible. It is clear, therefore, that this book should not be used as it is, but should serve as a basis for *local adaptation*. It should be noted, however, that the whole of this book may not necessarily require adaptation.[1] It may happen that only some parts of it need to be adapted to local conditions, health priorities, or different levels of trainees.

Adaptation is not always an easy task. The following guidelines have been prepared in the hope that public health administrators will find them useful when adapting this book for the use of their own CHWs. Adaptation is best done locally by people well acquainted with the prevailing situation, habits, and culture.

---

[1] This obviously does not apply to translation. Note that WHO encourages translation of its publications (particularly this one), and may provide a subsidy to organizations for doing so. See page 463 for more information.

2. Reviewing the role of CHWs in the national primary health care programme

The first step is to ascertain whether the country is ready to begin to train CHWs. To begin training CHWs before their place has been carefully planned and prepared in the health care system would be wrong. Left to themselves, without proper supervision and guidance, CHWs might very quickly lose the discipline and motivation needed to perform effectively tasks expected of them. The CHW is part of the health care delivery system. He is the peripheral member of the health team, which may include at the intermediate level the medical assistant or head nurse and at the next level the first physician. Thus, the CHW must not be trained or asked to work in isolation. His performance should be closely supervised.

The concept of community health work should be well understood and accepted by health personnel, community leaders, and the population if their support and participation are to be obtained. Lasting success cannot be achieved without their support and participation. They are essential for good cooperation between the three levels of the district health service: the village, where CHWs work; the health centre, usually run by a medical assistant; and the district or rural hospital, where a physician usually functions as the leader of the primary health care team.

3. Appointment of a working group

The Minister of Health could appoint a working group to adapt this book. The group should be small and should be chosen from among health administrators, public health physicians, nurses/ midwives, medical assistants in charge of rural health centres, physicians of rural hospitals, sanitarians, and community development personnel. The advice of other specialists should be obtained whenever necessary. The terms of reference of the group would be to follow the steps of the adaptation process indicated below.

4. The adaptation process

Deciding upon problems to be tackled by a CHW

Several factors will influence the decision as to which problems should be tackled by the CHW, the first of which is the role of the health team. Since the CHW is a member of that team, what he does will depend on what the others do. This is because in a health team the functions of all team members are complementary and related. For instance, the physician at a rural hospital performs Caesarean section, the medical assistant or public health nurse at a rural health centre inserts IUDs, while the CHW looks after normal pregnant women, treats their minor ailments, and refers the conditions he cannot deal with to the nurse or physician. Other factors that will determine the kind of work he undertakes are his previous education, the resources available, the stage of development of the country, the quality of supervision, and the referral system.

Because of the elementary nature of his education and training, the CHW should not be overloaded. Two or more community health workers may work in one community and share the work. For example, a male CHW may undertake environmental health work and a female worker may be made responsible for maternal and child health work.

Before selecting the areas that the CHWs will be expected to cover in their work, some criteria for the selection of topics will have to be established. In preparing this book, the topics were assigned priority according to the following criteria:

—demand from the public
—frequency of the disease or condition
—danger to the community
—danger to the individual

—technical feasibility of action by a CHW
—economic consequences of the problem.

The working group may decide to use these criteria in its selection. Furthermore, the 52 units in this book could serve as a framework or starting point for the working group to identify the problems to be tackled by CHWs.

Deciding upon skills authorized for a CHW

At what technical level should the CHW deal with each health problem? Consider the following questions:

(1) What role should a CHW play in maternity care, delivery, etc.?

(2) Should a CHW know how to detect albumin and sugar in urine? (If so, he should be given the means to do it.)

(3) What medicines can a CHW use or give?

(4) Should a CHW give injections? If so, which ones?

(5) Should a CHW be able to extract a tooth?

(6) Which form(s) should he regularly fill in?

Reviewing the job description of the CHW

The CHW's job and training will depend upon the problems he has to solve and upon his technical ability. To be sure that his training fits the tasks (task-oriented training), the working group should write (or rewrite) the CHW's job description, checking it against the list of agreed topics.

The job description will serve as a basis for defining learning objectives and preparing learning modules (see "Examples of learning modules", pages 443–450). It should be in the form of a list of tasks and duties, such as those given in the examples (see also Unit 49).

These examples of job descriptions may serve as a starting-point for the description of other tasks and duties a community may wish to entrust to a CHW.

Deletions and additions of topics will permit the CHW's job description to be tailored to the priorities of the population and of the health services. The new job description should be included at the beginning of the adapted national version of this book.

Identifying and deleting unsuitable units and selecting new topics to be added

This task will be easy if a job description has been drawn up for CHWs. The group can go through the units in this book and delete those that are not relevant to the job description. Similarly, any topics that are not covered in this book but are included in the job description can be added. It should be noted that all units that are retained should be adapted to local conditions and all new units should be written in the same way as those that are retained.

Adapting the units selected from this book

First the group may find that the titles of the units in this book are not suitable. For instance, Unit 18, "Planning a family", may need to be reworded, and some may prefer "Family planning", others "Birth spacing". The same may apply to other units.

The text itself may have to be reviewed and adapted so that the CHWs can easily understand it. It should correspond to local habits and beliefs and to regulations of the Ministry of Health. For example, the text of Unit 18, "Planning a family", should reflect national policy on family planning and should tell the CHWs which contraceptives they can recommend. Other units will need to be similarly adapted. Certain foods are easier to get in some countries than in others; consequently, they should be mentioned first in the unit on nutrition (see Unit 20). The text should describe how to make the best use of the common foods and how to supplement them, when necessary, by other foodstuffs that people can easily get and afford.

Annex 1 lists and recommends 22 essential *medicines* or drugs and gives their generic names, but national health authorities may prefer other names better known to their health workers and the public. Dosage and packaging may vary from one country to another, and therefore the list should be carefully revised and modified. Other essential medicines or drugs may be added, especially when they are known to be effective, are safe, cheap, widely used, and included in the essential drugs list officially recommended by the government. They should be selected very carefully in order to avoid misuse, abuse, and unnecessary expense.

Attention should also be paid to the *drawings* to be included in the adapted version of this book. For instance, pigs should not be shown in drawings in countries where their meat is not eaten. Injection techniques should not be illustrated in countries where the CHWs are not allowed to give injections. Drawings that reflect national characteristics and the national scene will be preferable to those in this book.

In many countries there are official regulations and instructions with which health workers must comply; when applicable, they should be included (after revision, if necessary) in the national version in order not to contradict the official authorities of the country.

In order to promote the development of primary health care, all parts of this guide may be freely adapted, translated, or used in any form for non-profit-making purposes. Prior permission to do so need not be obtained from the World Health Organization, but appropriate reference should be made to this source.

Presenting and detailing the new problems added

If new units are to be added to the adapted version of this book, they should be written and presented in the same way as the units that are retained.

In writing up the learning content the group should imagine itself in the position of the CHW who is intelligent, motivated and full of goodwill but who has limited education and training. The instructions should be clear, easy to follow, and written in a simple way. By following those instructions the CHW should be able to carry out effective and safe action. He should be guided to refer any problem that is beyond his competence.

It should be noted that writing instructions clearly and in a simple way is not always easy. One effective way is to make a flow-chart of the problem by breaking it up into several steps. An example of this approach is given below for the problem of dealing with fractures.

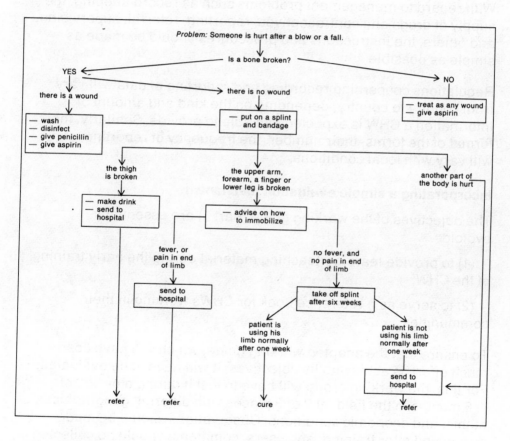

Thus, when the CHW suspects a fracture, he should be able to find guidance in his book on what to do. He should also be able to remember what he has learned during his training and should be satisfied that he has taken the right decision. The same process can be applied to any other problem.

The text should be kept to a minimum. It should give prominence to preventive measures and official regulations and instructions. It should be illustrated by simple drawings that any CHW can easily understand. A local artist could be asked to help with illustrations.

Care should be taken to use the list of essential medicines already agreed upon, and any new product that is needed should belong to the list of essential drugs agreed upon by the Ministry of Health. With regard to management problems such as record-keeping, the supply of drugs and contraceptives, reporting, referral, supervision, and others, the instructions and procedures should be made as simple as possible.

Regulations concerning recording and reporting of data will vary from country to country, depending on the kind and amount of information a CHW is expected and able to provide. Similarly, the format of the forms, their number, the frequency of reporting, etc. will vary with local conditions.

Incorporating a simple evaluation mechanism

The objectives of the working guide (Part 1) are essentially twofold:

(1) to provide learning/teaching material during the early training of the CHW;

(2) to serve as a reference book for CHWs working in their communities.

To ensure that the adapted working guide, which will have cost much effort, is achieving its objectives, it will have to be evaluated. For this, the working group will have to test it during a period of 4–6 months in the field, at 2 or 3 places with different geographical, ethnic, and economic conditions. Observations should be made during and after training, and users' comments should be collected by means of a previously prepared questionnaire, designed to find out:

- how useful the working guide has been
- where it has failed

- what difficulties have been experienced in its use
- what corrections or modifications are required
- what additions or deletions are required
- what changes, if any, are required in the content, presentation, drawings, etc.

When collected and analysed, these comments and suggestions will help in the production of an improved new edition of the working guide. Further re-evaluations along the same lines should lead in a few years to a working guide well adapted to local conditions, serving as a valuable tool for CHWs.

5. How to use this book

As mentioned earlier, this book can be used in two ways within the national primary health care programme: as material for training and as a reference book. When used for training, it is intended mainly for CHWs. The first page of each learning unit gives the learning objectives. This is for the benefit of both the CHW and his trainer. Stated as tasks, the learning objectives indicate what a CHW will be able to do at the end of training that he could not do before. The learning objectives should also enable trainee CHWs to understand better their learning activities and why they need to be trained.

On the second page of each unit is a simple explanation of the topic of the unit. For instance, "pregnancy", "intestinal worms", "venereal diseases" are all technical terms the meaning of which is obvious to an educated health worker, but, most probably, not to a CHW at the beginning of training.
Then follow a few pages of learning content, illustrated by simple drawings, which describe how health problems can be prevented or dealt with, and the procedures the CHW should follow: what to look for, check, ask and do.

In his daily work the CHW will have to use a few medicines or drugs, take temperatures, apply bandages and possibly give certain injections. Special instructions on how to do these tasks are given in the annexes to this book; these will have to be adapted to local requirements by the national health authorities.

Although the guide is intended primarily for CHWs, it will also prove useful to all those responsible for the training of community health workers (physicians, medical assistants, nurses, sanitarians, administrators). As mentioned before, the teachers should be familiar with its contents: job description of the CHW, learning objectives corresponding to each unit, and the annexes. Annex 3, which shows anatomical diagrams, is intended mainly for the CHWs' trainers. Some of these diagrams may be too complex and difficult for CHWs while others may be inappropriate; the situation will vary from country to country. The drawings may nevertheless be useful to trainers and can serve as models for their blackboard drawings.

The CHWs should keep their working guide very carefully as it will be a precious companion to which they can refer whenever necessary, e.g., to check the action they should take in case of a problem, the dose of a medicine, or other instructions and regulations. The content of the working guide represents basic training material, which must be built on and continuously improved. CHWs should be asked to note in the book the results of their experiences, the advice of their supervisors, and additional information they receive from the health services.

6. Translation [1]

The working document will be fully adapted only when it is translated into local languages. This is a difficult and delicate task that should only be entrusted to the most skilled translator. The translation should be revised by health officials who are fully aware of local diseases and conditions, health and medical terminology,

---

[1] See footnote 1 on page 451. See also page 463.

and local usages, practices, and names. A physician might be specially appointed by the ministry of health or the working group to be responsible for the translation and publication. One need hardly stress the importance of accuracy, since an error in translation or printing could have serious consequences.

7. Printing

Once it has been adapted and translated, the national working guide should be issued in a format that CHWs can use easily during their training, and later for reference and for continuing education. The book should be able to stand up to the hard conditions of community work, and it should also have space for new information to be added. A loose-leaf format would permit new material to be prepared for later training sessions, but it might be more expensive and less hard-wearing and there is a serious risk that pages may be lost or new material not inserted.

This book has three parts, of which only the first, entitled "Working guide", is intended for CHWs. The second part, "Guidelines for training community health workers" is meant for trainers of CHWs, and the third "Guidelines for adapting this book", is of concern to public health administrators and trainers. Since only the first part should be given to CHWs, it seems logical that it should be printed separately from the two other parts. The annexes on medicines and techniques should be included with Part 1.

The first edition of the adapted working guide might be printed cheaply for field testing. Feedback from field testing would make it possible to correct errors, modify the text or its presentation, and add important comments or material. This would improve the second edition, make it more valuable and justify its wide distribution.

SUBSIDIES FOR TRANSLATION

Financial assistance may be available to organizations (not individuals) wishing to translate, print and distribute WHO publications in languages other than those normally used by the various offices of WHO (that is, languages other than Arabic, Chinese, English, French, German, Portuguese, Russian or Spanish). The assistance would cover only a proportion of the costs involved in translation, printing and distribution.

WHO will consider giving such assistance under the following circumstances. (1) The WHO publication concerned should be highly relevant to health activities in the area where the language is used. (2) The language should be one that is widely read, not merely spoken. (3) The translation should be necessary because a large proportion of the health workers to whom the WHO publication is addressed are unable to read it in any language in which it already exists. (4) The applicant body, which could, for instance, be a government department, professional organization or commercial publisher, should be able to ensure translation and printing of a reasonably high standard and should have access to adequate facilities for distributing the work.

A fully detailed application should be addressed to the WHO regional office, as shown below, corresponding to the country where the applicant body is located. Preference will be given to applications from the countries mentioned, which are among those listed by the United Nations as "most seriously affected" or "least developed".

Regional Office for Africa, P.O. Box No. 6, Brazzaville, Congo: Benin, Botswana, Burkina Faso, Burundi, Cape Verde, Cameroon, Central African Republic, Chad, Comoros, Côte d'Ivoire, Ethiopia, Gambia, Ghana, Guinea, Guinea-Bissau, Kenya, Lesotho, Madagascar, Malawi, Mali, Mauritania, Mozambique, Niger, Rwanda, Senegal, Sierra Leone, Uganda, United Republic of Tanzania.

Regional Office for South-East Asia, World Health House, Indraprastha Estate, Mahatma Gandhi Road, New Delhi—110 002, India: Bangladesh, Bhutan, Burma, India, Maldives, Nepal, Sri Lanka.

Regional Office for the Eastern Mediterranean, P.O. Box 1517, Alexandria—21511, Egypt: Afghanistan, Democratic Yemen, Egypt, Pakistan, Somalia, Sudan, Yemen.

Regional Office for the Western Pacific, P.O. Box 2932, Manila 2801, Philippines: Democratic Kampuchea, Lao People's Democratic Republic, Samoa.

SOCIAL SCIENCE LIBRARY

Building

WHO publications may be obtained, direct or through booksellers, from:

ALGERIA: Entreprise nationale du Livre (ENAL), 3 bd Zirout Youce, ALGIERS

ARGENTINA: Carlos Hirsch, SRL, Florida 165, Galerías Güemes, Escritorio 453/465, BUENOS AIRES

AUSTRALIA: Hunter Publications, 58A Gipps Street, COLLINGWOOD, VIC 3066 — Australian Government Publishing Service *(Mail order sales)*, P.O. Box 84, CANBERRA A.C.T. 2601; *or over the counter from:* Australian Government Publishing Service Booshops *at:* 70 Alinga Street, CANBERRA CITY A.C.T. 2600; 294 Adelaide Street, BRISBANE, Queensland 4000; 347 Swanston Street, MELBOURNE, VIC 3000; 309 Pitt Street, SYDNEY, N.S.W. 2000; Mt Newman House, 200 St. George's Terrace, PERTH, WA 6000; Industry House, 12 Pirie Street, ADELAIDE, SA 5000; 156–162 Macquarie Street, HOBART, TAS 7000 — R. Hill & Son Ltd., 608 St. Kilda Road, MELBOURNE, VIC 3004; Lawson House, 10–12 Clark Street, CROW'S NEST, NSW 2065

AUSTRIA: Gerold & Co., Graben 31, 1011 VIENNA I

BANGLADESH: The WHO Programme Coordinator, G.P.O Box 250, DHAKA 5

BELGIUM: *For books:* Office International de Librairie s.a., avenue Marnix 30, 1050 BRUSSELS. *For periodicals and subscriptions:* Office International des Périodiques, avenue Louise 485, 1050 BRUSSELS — *Subscriptions to World Health only:* Jean de Lannoy, 202 avenue du Roi, 1060 BRUSSELS

BHUTAN: *see* India, WHO Regional Office

BOTSWANA: Botsalo Books (Pty) Ltd., P.O. Box 1532, GABORONE

BRAZIL: Biblioteca Regional de Medicina OMS/OPS, Sector de Publicações, Caixa Postal 20.381, Vila Clementino, 04023 SÃO PAULO, S.P.

BURMA: *see* India, WHO Regional Office

CANADA: Canadian Public Health Association, 1335 Carling Avenue, Suite 210, OTTAWA, Ont. K1Z 8N8. (Tel: (613) 725–3769. Telex: 21–053–3841)

CHINA: China National Publications Import & Export Corporation, P.O. Box 88, BEIJING (PEKING)

DEMOCRATIC PEOPLE'S REPUBLIC OF KOREA: *see* India, WHO Regional Office

DENMARK: Munksgaard Export and Subscription Service, Nørre Søgade 35, 1370 COPENHAGEN K (Tel: + 45 1 12 85 70)

FIJI: The WHO Programme Coordinator, P.O. Box 113, SUVA

FINLAND: Akateeminen Kirjakauppa, Keskuskatu 2, 00101 HELSINKI 10

FRANCE: Librairie Arnette, 2 rue Casimir-Delavigne, 75006 PARIS

GERMAN DEMOCRATIC REPUBLIC: Buchhaus Leipzig, Postfach 140, 701 LEIPZIG

GERMANY FEDERAL REPUBLIC OF: Govi-Verlag GmbH, Ginnheimerstrasse 20, Postfach 5360, 6236 ESCHBORN — Buchhandlung Alexander Horn, Friedrichstrasse 39, Postfach 3340, 6200 WIESBADEN

GHANA: Fides Enterprises, P.O. Box 1628, ACCRA

GREECE: G.C. Eleftheroudakis S.A., Librairie internationale, rue Nikis 4, ATHENS (T. 126)

HONG KONG: Hong Kong Government Information Services, Beaconsfield House, 6th Floor, Queen's Road, Central, VICTORIA

HUNGARY: Kultura, P.O.B. 149, BUDAPEST 62

INDIA: WHO Regional Office for South-East Asia, World Health House, Indraprastha Estate, Mahatma Gandhi Road, NEW DELHI 110002

INDONESIA: P.T. Kalman Media Pusaka, Pusat Perdagangan Senen, Block 1, 4th Floor, P.O. Box 3433/Jkt, JAKARTA

IRAN (ISLAMIC REPUBLIC OF): Iran University Press, 85 Park Avenue, P.O. Box 54/551, TEHERAN

IRELAND: TDC Publishers, 12 North Frederick Street, DUBLIN 1 (Tel: 744835–749677)

ISRAEL: Heiliger & Co., 3 Nathan Strauss Street, JERUSALEM 94227

ITALY: Edizioni Minerva Medica, Corso Bramante 83–85, 10126 TURIN; Via Lamarmora 3, 20100 MILAN; Via Spallanzani 9, 00161 ROME

JAPAN: Maruzen Co. Ltd., P.O. Box 5050, TOKYO International, 100–31

JORDAN: Jordan Book Centre Co. Ltd., University Street, P.O. Box 301 (Al-Jubeiha), AMMAN

KUWAIT: The Kuwait Bookshops Co. Ltd., Thunayan Al-Ghanem Bldg, P.O. Box 2942, KUWAIT

LAOS PEOPLE'S DEMOCRATIC REPUBLIC: The WHO Programme Coordinator, P.O. Box 343, VIENTIANE

LUXEMBOURG: Librairie du Centre, 49 bd Royal, LUXEMBOURG

MALAWI: Malawi Book Service, P.O. Box 30044, Chichiri, BLANTYRE 3

A/1/86